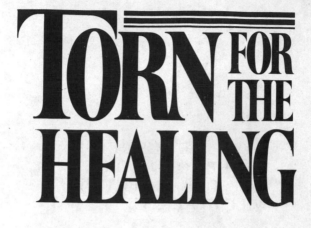

"COME, LET US RETURN
TO THE LORD. FOR HE
HAS TORN US, BUT HE
WILL HEAL US."

Hosea 6:1 & 2

TORN FOR THE HEALING

C. Brandon Rimmer

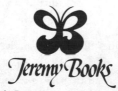

Jeremy Books

5624 Lincoln Drive, Minneapolis, Minnesota 55436

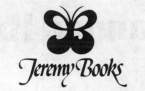

Jeremy Books

5624 Lincoln Drive, Minneapolis, Minnesota 55436

INTRODUCTION

At the edge of Buckley, Washington, near the northwest foot of Mt. Rainier is a school for retarded children, the Rainier School. It consists of many buildings, some single story, some two and three story, buildings spread out over many green and grassy acres. I was in one of the central buildings in the office of Charles B. Sweigard, M.D., waiting for him to return from a staff meeting. I looked around the room. A lovely portrait of a lovely woman caught my eye immediately. It was a painting of Beth, Dr. Sweigard's present wife, done by her gifted artist brother, John Soli. Artistic ability runs in the family—Beth's pictures are also becoming known across the country.

Behind the picture there were books that one would expect to find on the desk of a practicing pediatrician. I picked one up and looked at the charts and statistics that covered its pages. They were no longer just statistics to me. They had been changed from statistics to people as I had wandered around the institution. Mrs. Frogh had graciously escorted me through Holly Hall, the part of the complex for which she was responsible.

In Holly there were men with bodies that were young adult, but with minds of very limited intelligence, minds so young that they weren't intelligent enough to learn to speak. Worse, some were inclined to self-destruct, and they had crash helmets locked on their heads so that during a seizure, they couldn't beat their brains out against the wall or the floor.

Mrs. Frogh spoke to them in a kindly manner, and some smiled at her. Several of the patients wanted to touch me. I let them do it; they meant me no harm but were only curious. They had the kind of curiosity one expects from an eighteen-month-old child. The color and texture of my blue-grey coat intrigued them.

The place was neat, clean, and well run by any standards, but it was still "a place." It was of necessity an institution. It had been built and was being run for children who were mentally retarded, and there was no way that you could color that picture happy. The staff members were obviously humane, but still no matter how you spelled it, it came out depressing.

When Dr. Sweigard came back into his office a patient followed him. The contrast between the doctor and the patient was striking. The doctor was tall, grey-haired and good-looking; the patient was about fourteen years old, with a slightly twisted body and a badly twisted mind. Chuck Sweigard explained to the patient that he had company in his office waiting for him, and he told the boy to come back and see him the same time the next day. By speaking slowly and with great patience, he was able to make the child understand, and we watched as the boy hobbled away willingly enough, happy to look forward to the following day.

Chuck Sweigard speaks to his patients with great kindness. There is a special reason for his kindness. Dr. Sweigard has been a patient in mental institutions, one who was incorrectly diagnosed and unjustly incarcerated. The experience added up to years of private hell in three different asylums. He has been on the wrong end of the medication and he knows what it is like. This book is his story.

C. Brandon Rimmer

This is a real story about real people. The medical reports are copied from the originals. However, some names, dates, and places have been changed to protect those involved.

CHAPTER ONE

PART I

STOCKTON STATE HOSPITAL
510 East Magnolia St.
Stockton, California 95202

30 Aug. 65 RT-1

IDENTIFICATION: This 35-year-old, white married physician, the father of five, was committed as mentally ill on August 30, in his first state hospitalization.

RECOMMENDATION: Patient will be transferred to LPNI on 6-31-65 and hospital transportation will be necessary to effect this transfer. Patient has been passive in preparation for transfer and should present no problem in transportation at this time.

The state car exited from highway 101 in downtown San Francisco and drove west on Fell Street toward the east end of the Golden Gate Park. The driver kept to the right until he reached Stanyan St. and then turned left. The white-coated attendants sat in the front of the grey car. Dr. Charles Sweigard sat in the back, separated from the men in front of him by a heavy, reinforced wire screen. There were no door handles on the inside of the rear doors, nor could the windows be rolled down.

The car climbed steeply to Parnassus Ave. and turned right up the hill. As they turned, Chuck noticed a small food store near the southwest corner. He was to become better acquainted with that place later. At the top of the hill, just before they reached the Langley Porter Neuropsychiatric Institute, the car turned left into a curved alley that circled behind the building. As they entered the alley, the garrish multistoried building was on their right. On their left was a highly shielded play yard for children. The fence went twenty feet into the air and was interwoven so that little could be seen through it. But things could be heard. Some child was screaming at the top of his lungs.

At the back of the hospital the driver stopped the car. He and the other attendant climbed out, and both of them stood by the back door of the car as Chuck exited. They were taking no chances. The Stockton Hospital diagnosis had been "Schizophrenic Reaction, Paranoid Type." That meant one thing to them. The patient was unpredictable.

The entrance to Langley Porter differed from the entrance to Stockton in that as they went into LPNI, the two huge doors slammed shut behind them. At Stockton there had been only one door.

Langley Porter had been easy to enter, the two muscular attendants had seen to that. Chuck's problem was just to find a simple answer to a simple question.

"How do I get out?"

He had a feeling that it was not going to be easy. The psychiatrist back at Stockton had not cared for Chuck and the dislike had shown through the whole proceeding. The diagnosis had been vicious and unwarranted. It was a great way to put somebody under—Schizophrenic paranoids rarely get well.

THE LANGLEY PORTER NEUROPSYCHI-
ATRIC INSTITUTE
401 Parnassus Avenue
San Francisco, California 94122

DISCHARGE SUMMARY
January 17, 1966

Sweigard, Charles, B., Jr.
LPNI No. 6928

DATE OF ADMISSION: August 31, 1965

DATE OF DISCHARGE: January 17, 1966

REASON FOR ADMISSION: Fear of dying and religious preoccupations.

REFERRED BY: Dr. Winkler, Staff Psychiatrist, Stockton State Hospital

TREATMENT AND COURSE: He received Tofranil to doses of 225 mg. daily for two weeks and Prolixin, to doses of 5 mg. q.i.d. His discharge medica-

*tions were Tofranil, 150 mg. daily, Prolixin, 2.5 mg.
q.i.d. and Cogentin, 2 mg. daily.*

31 Aug 65
SAN FRANCISCO

The room at Langley Porter had twelve beds in
it. Six were on the left of the hall door, and six
more, across from each other, were on the right.
The wall on the left had a doorless opening in the
center which led into the showers and the toilets.
Chuck was to spend a lot of time in there.

His admission was followed by three days of apparent disregard, but he knew that he was under
observation. He did a little observing of his own.
The men in the room with him were in various
stages of insanity, but they all had one thing in
common. They couldn't walk properly. Their coordination had been affected somehow and their awkward shuffling was slightly grotesque. He wondered
what it was that they had in common.

The answer to his question was on the way. He
had been committed at a time when Langley Porter
was handing out a drug called Prolixin like it was
candy. It had the effect of crippling the ability to
think independently, so that the mind of the patient
could be worked on by the psychiatrist. It had the
additional effect of hurting the body.

On the fourth day Chuck was approached by a
nurse. She was a hard-looking woman who, under
other circumstances, might not have been. She
could afford neither sympathy nor understanding

at the moment. She was doing her job—the most unpleasant part of it. She was giving drugs to a doctor. Unlike most patients, the doctor would want to know what he was taking. The connection between Prolixin and the side effects of the twisted back, the sore muscles and the shuffling walk, would be guessed immediately. Chuck was surrounded by horrible examples.

She spoke to him in as authoritative a manner as she dared. "Here's your medication, Doctor."

"What is it?"

She told him.

"What does it do?"

She told him that too.

"No thank you." He said it quietly but firmly, and there was a note of finality in his voice. She looked at him for a minute, shrugged and turned away. She still had the pills in her hand.

PART II

RT-1 (Summary continued)

COURSE & TREATMENT: Patient has steadfastly refused to accept tranquilizing medication. He has a desperate need to deny mental illness, feels that there is nothing wrong with him, that he does not require hospitalization and that his present plight is just another obstacle to him in his godly approach to earthlings. . .

7 Sept 65
SAN FRANCISCO

One of the attendants stuck his head in the door and motioned to Chuck to follow him. "This way please, Doctor."

Chuck got up from the bed on which he had been sitting. It was against the hospital rules to lie down during the day. The time was soon coming when he would have too much pain to keep walking, and too much pain when he sat down, but the rule would still hold, no lying down during the day time.

He followed the attendant down the hall to a small room that they both entered. The attendant closed the door behind them. Chuck heard it lock. Inside the room there was another attendant waiting. His muscular arms were folded across his considerable chest. The young psychiatrist who was in charge of Chuck's case was there, and so was the nurse who had tried to give him his pills. This time there were no pills. She had a hypodermic needle in her hand that seemed to Chuck to be about the right size for a small horse.

The psychiatrist broke the silence. "One way or another, Dr. Sweigard, you're going to take this medicine. You can put up a fight if you want to, but you don't stand a chance. We've had lots of practice."

Chuck looked at them. He didn't have a chance. Two muscle men plus a doctor and a nurse.

"This is a chemical lobotomy and you know it."

"Dr. Sweigard, you may call it anything you please, but you'll take the medicine. You have been judged legally insane. I have been put in charge of your case."

"Are you going to put that mixed dosage of all those drugs in one cheek?"

"Yes. And next time you're handed medication ordered by your doctor give yourself a break and take it."

There was nothing that could be done.

Chuck undid his belt. It was to be months before he would walk again without pain and without abnormal movement. Worse, he was going to have to fight for his individuality and his personal integrity. He was going to have to fight the psychiatrist, the environment and the drugs, and keep convincing himself that what had happened had happened and what he had seen he had seen. It was not going to be easy.

CHAPTER TWO

PART I

20 Aug 65 RT-1: PRESENT ILLNESS: Apparently there has been increasing friction between his wife and himself over the years of their marriage. The wife has been sexually frigid, neurotic, demanding and has been inclined to be a social climber and live beyond their means`, had never wished to settle in Modesto and never let her husband forget this.

(Approximately fifteen months earlier)

9 June 64
MODESTO

Chuck came to the Tuesday morning breakfast table bleary-eyed. An emergency had taken place at two in the morning and it had robbed him of his sleep. Nothing robbed him of his patience and kindness. He didn't have any of either, and you can't take from a man what he doesn't have. He broke the silence that had settled over his wife and children when he had come into the room.

"I see that you have outdone yourself again this morning for a large and satisfying breakfast; Grape

Nuts or Corn Flakes with canned peaches. Congratulations on your cuisine."

His wife, Cathy responded in kind. "If you don't want to eat it, you know what to do with it."

Chuck changed from criticizing the food to criticizing the way she was dressed. "I see you're in your shorts again."

Shorts were very becoming to her. Cathy did not look like the mother of five children. Her stomach was flat, her legs lean and well tanned. Chuck continued. "How can you go play tennis when the house is unkept?"

"Because the woman who cleans it will not be here until tomorrow."

The children sat as silently as they always did when their parents were fighting. That made for a lot of silence.

"You can't keep the house looking decent by having it straightened out once a week."

"Then give me enough money to have her come every day."

Chuck put down his spoon and looked at his cereal bowl. He never had liked cold cereal anyway. "Listen, when we lived in Tokyo and I was an Air Force doctor, we could have 'Mama-san' for twenty dollars a month. She and her helpers could clean, cook and wipe the baby while you sat around like a queen. We're not in Tokyo any more. Servants cost money in Modesto."

"Everything costs money in Modesto and there's nothing here worth buying."

"You buy tennis lessons."

"The next thing I know, you'll accuse me of buying the Pro."

"It would serve him right if you did."

Cathy turned white. "Go to work and earn your dollar and twenty-five cents for the day."

PART II

RT-1 PRESENT ILLNESS: In addition to this domestic pressure, patient was faced with an inordinately heavy pediatric burden which grew rapidly and he was under the stress of proving himself to be acceptable for future partnership in the medical group.

9 June 64 Cont.
MODESTO

Chuck left the kitchen table, his half-eaten breakfast ignored, picked up his black bag and walked out of the hall door and into the patio that was between the house and the street. The patio was enclosed by a six-foot wall and fence and the gate was next to the side of the garage. He went through the gate and the three car garage was on his right. Across the street there was a new "For Sale" sign placed in the front yard of the house opposite his.

He knew why it was there. The house had belonged to a colleague, a doctor who had been trying to make it into the same medical group that Chuck was trying to enter. It was not easy to get in. Every doctor who tried to come into the group came in on a two year probation arrangement. If the new doctor grossed four times his salary he was usually voted into membership, but the money wasn't the only criterion. There was a great deal of pride taken in the quality of the medicine practiced by the group. Mediocre work was not acceptable. Mediocrity had been his neighbor's problem. He had been a surgeon, but not a very good one, and he'd realized that he wasn't making the grade with his peers. That led to drinking, which led to drinking on the job. That led to a shaky hand. That led to a warning to get ready to leave the group. That led to his wife's filing for divorce. That led to acute depression. That led to a wild ride southbound on highway 99, at an ever increasing speed until his car couldn't make the curves. He rolled to his death.

The widow got the insurance as the divorce wasn't final. The only other thing that might have prevented payment was solid evidence of suicide. Such evidence was hard to come by. It was true that the alcoholic content of his blood at the time of the accident had been phenomonal, but you can't prove that drunk driving is suicide even if you are sure that it is. So the insurance company had to pay off. That insurance, plus the money that would come from the sale of the house would let the widow take herself and her children back East to her former home and do it in style. But, in style, or in poverty, it was unpleasant business. So too, sometimes, was marriage to a doctor. Chuck would have bet a hundred dollars that if the widow married again it wouldn't be to another M.D.

He put his bag in the back of his sports coupe, climbed into the driver's seat, started the motor and backed out into the street. He headed north to the east bound street he needed. It had a bridge that crossed the creek on his right, the creek that was the east boundary line of the subdivision that included his home. The north end of it was a park deeded to the city. It was a pretty park, with sloping green lawns that undulated down to the edge of the creek.

As he drove, he mused about his own position. His gross was rapidly approaching the desired figure, and his medicine was good. He knew it. He also let it be known. This latter point raised a problem with his colleagues. He didn't keep his mouth shut about his good or anyone else's bad. When he saw poor medicine he said so, and some of his criticisms had been brutal. When it came time to vote him in or out, there would be a lot of the younger doctors hoping he'd lose; but the important votes were cast by the older men, and they liked his medicine and his income. If the newer doctors hated him, that was tough.

Also of help to Chuck was the fact that the group was losing a senior partner who had no love for Charles B. Sweigard, M.D. The partner was an older man, a psychiatrist, and he had been the butt of a couple of Chuck's sarcastic remarks. The remarks were not based on ignorance; psychiatry was an area about which Sweigard knew quite a little. He'd graduated from the University of Pennsylvania Medical School, and they were heavy on psychiatry for all students, including pediatricians. Chuck thought the psychiatrist a quack and made no bones about it, but the dislike that this had generated was not going to trouble the waters. The shrink was leaving the group and had accepted a job as a psychiatrist at the state hospital in Stockton. That would take him out of Chuck's life, as far as Chuck knew.

He turned his car to the right again. That morning he had no patients in the City Hospital and so he turned south toward the Scenic. Parking at the Scenic Hospital was a little difficult, the doctor parking spaces at the north end had been crowded out by people parking for the county health department. He slid into a space that was only mildly illegal and taking his bag out of the car trunk, went into the hospital.

As soon as he was in his professional environment, all the childishness that characterized his relationship with his family disappeared and a mode of operation that impressed people took its place. He was comparatively young, good looking, prematurely grey, and he exuded confidence. The nurses practically melted. In about fifteen minutes he was through at Scenic, had re-entered his car and was headed for the Medical Group building. He was glad he didn't have to drive past that building and go on to the Doctor's Hospital. It so happened that he had no patients in that facility that morning. It was an unusual day. He had patients in only one hospital. He didn't want to drive to the east side of town. It wasn't that he didn't like the Doctor's hos-

pital. He enjoyed its thick red carpets and its ingra-
tiating and ubiquitous personnel; it was just that
the Doctor's hospital was too close to the Racquet
Club and his tennis-playing wife.

At the Medical Group building, he had no trouble parking. In that parking lot, each doctor had his
name printed in black letters on a yellow background in each one of about fifty spaces reserved
for the doctors in the group. The one marked
Charles B. Sweigard was empty, as it should be. He
parked in it, retrieved his bag and walked in the
southeast entrance marked "Staff only." He turned
left once he was inside. The pediatrics department
was on the first floor, in the southwest corner of the
building.

PART III

14 June 64
MODESTO

Chuck sat in church listening to the minister
with only half an ear. The part of the Episcopalian
service that Chuck enjoyed, the music, was over
and the sermon had begun. He liked the music and
enjoyed singing. His voice was a pleasant baritone
and fit into the choir easily. He'd been part of a
choir for as long as he could remember. Back in
Bethlehem, Pennsylvania, where he had been
raised, he had been in a child's choir and then later,
had been a boy soprano and soloist in the chancel

choir. All of this experience had taught him to read music, and enabled him to sing almost anywhere he pleased.

Bored by the sermon, Chuck turned through the church calendar reading about the events of the week. One item in particular caught and held his attention. It concerned a young woman who ran a mission for drug addicts in downtown San Francisco. She was to speak that Sunday evening in the parish hall of the Episcopal church. Chuck decided to go hear her.

Like all pediatricians, indeed like all doctors, he was running into more and more abuse of drugs as a patient problem. Even in Modesto drug abuse was assuming serious and growing proportions. The statistics were frightening. It might be worth his time to hear what the young lady had to say.

When he got to the meeting, he was surprised by the size of the crowd. Generally, the Sunday service was poorly attended, but this speaker and this subject had increased the attendance. Among the non-church-members present were half a dozen doctors whom he knew. They were probably there for the same reason he was—patients' abuse of drugs.

When the speaker began her talk she got immediate and undivided attention. She was statuesque, a striking brunette and a gifted speaker. In addition to all this, was another factor that attracted Chuck the moment she started talking. Soon he realized that it was the laughter in her eyes and the joy in her voice. In Chuck's world there was too little of either of these.

She said that she had become an addict at the age of ten and had "mainlined" for eight years. She had been hospitalized with an O.D. three times and had almost died each time. As she talked there was a certain skepticism in the room, particularly from the doctors present. Their skepticism was based on experience. There are certain signs— physical, mental, emotional; signs that do not disappear from an addict, not for years (if they ever leave) and the speaker was without those tell-tale characteristics.

She could feel the unbelief in the room, so she took off her jacket exposing her arms. They were tracked from one end to the other. They had been mercilessly scarred. She hadn't always used a needle. The unbelief in the room began to diminish. It diminished further as she talked about addiction. She knew things about heroin, $C_{21} H_{23} O_5 N$, things that people don't usually know unless they are doctors or educated addicts. She fielded questions from the floor easily and talked from an impressive level of experience. When she felt that the skepticism had been dispelled, she told the story of her conversion.

"I'm not the product of the ghetto. My family were educated, well-to-do people who had in me a daughter who turned viciously rebellious at the age of ten. They didn't know why, and I don't know why. We battled for eight years, and then, with a sense of failure, humiliation, and faint hope, they signed me over, just before my eighteenth birthday, to a Christian boarding school in the midwest.

"The school was in the 'toolies', there was no way for me to get a fix, no way at all. There weren't any drugs at the school and there wasn't anything else anywhere near the fenced-in school. For me it meant 'cold turkey'.

"They put me in a room with a very lovely girl. She was beautiful, quiet and unassuming. Her unfailing courtesy drove me nuts. Finally I was so stir crazy I attacked her. When she was scratched, bleeding and had half the clothes torn off her she was lying on the floor at my feet. I asked her, 'What am I going to have to do to you? Why don't you fight back?'

"Her reply was the most startling that I've ever heard in my life. She said, 'Because I love you.'

"How could you love me?"

"Because if I'd been through what you've been through, I might be worse than you. It's not me who's different, it's Jesus in me who's different. That's why I love you."

"I heard the words 'I love you' before, but under different circumstances and with a different meaning. This time, something in me clicked and I knew I was going to listen. I helped her up off the floor and she started talking to me as we sat side by side on her bed. She told me that God loved me, that Jesus Christ was God's Son and that He had died for my sins. That He rose from the dead, and that He was in the room with us. She told me that if I would turn my life and myself over to Him, that He would start living in me and change my life.

"I thought about it for a while and then I got down on my knees and did it, and for the first time in my life that I can clearly remember, I cried my heart out.

"My roommate helped me undress and go to

bed and I cried myself to sleep, but the crying changed into a good kind of crying, crying that comes from relief. I slept for four hours. When I woke up, I was conscious of the Lord's presence in the room. I was conscious of something else too. All—and I mean all—the characteristics of my addiction were gone, all but the tracks on my arms. It was as though I had never taken heroin in my life."

The room was quiet, so quiet that the tall clock in the entrance hall could be heard slowly ticking. She started talking again.

"I've gone back to San Francisco. I've rented a store front, some friends helped me raise the money, and I just talk to kids who are hooked and tell them about Jesus and what He has done for me. There are a lot more stories now, just like mine. Jesus saves, Jesus heals, the Lord is alive."

Charles B. Sweigard, M.D. sat stunned. It was the same Gospel story he'd heard when he went to the Christian and Missionary Alliance Sunday meetings with his grandmother back in Pennsylvania, but nobody had hit the "saw dust trail" who had ight years of heroin tracks down both arms. Something had happened to this girl that couldn't happen, but it had happened. He sat silently, wishing to God it could happen to him. He didn't have the heroin habit, he avoided drugs like the plague, but there were other things. There was that night in Hong Kong . . .

CHAPTER THREE

PART I

RT-1 PRESENT ILLNESS: (Continued) About one year ago, the patient became increasingly interested in religion and his detachment became noticeable and grew from that point . . .

15 Sept 64
MODESTO

Tuesday the fifteenth had been one of Chuck's worst days. He was glad it was almost over. Nothing had gone as it should have gone, and he was exhausted. He had raised the level of his practice, and that increase had made him incredibly busy. The pressure of the practice was added to by the fact that he had made so many enemies among the doctors that he didn't dare make a mistake. He had to practice flawless medicine at a breakneck pace and he was coming apart at the center.

Things at home hadn't helped. Sex had been perfunctory but it was worse than that now. Cathy had told him that she'd do her wifely duties when required, but she'd appreciate it if he'd keep it at a minimum. It meant nothing to her.

His rapport with his children was no better. It was an anomaly that a doctor who had chosen pediatrics because of his affinity for children and his ability to handle them, should find himself at total odds with his own sons and daughters. There was a wall between him and them, and he didn't know how to get over it.

Also, the thing for which he had aimed had lost its appeal. What difference did it make if he was accepted into the Medical Group? He didn't see any strikingly happy lives among the senior partners. On the whole they seemed a rather unhappy lot. What was the point of it all?

On top of all this there was one other factor. There was the face of the converted dope addict, the tall, beautiful girl from San Francisco. He couldn't forget her eyes nor the undercurrent of peace that ran through her words.

Ever since he had heard her testimony, he had tried to stay awake during the church service and listen to the Sunday morning sermons, but he'd gotten nothing from them that would help. The correct words were all there, the name of the Father, Son and Holy Spirit filled the liturgy of each service, but he could feel no life and he got no encouragement. It was as though the girl from San Francisco belonged to another world.

He had had a bite of evening supper in the cafeteria that was in the center of the first floor of the Doctor's Hospital. The food hadn't been particularly appetizing, but then Cathy's Tuesday evening meal might have been worse. At least he hadn't had to go home and sit through the family meal, a meal that would have been punctuated by endless and pointless bickering.

He had left the hospital dining room as though he really did have some place to go and walked briskly toward the parking lot where doctors parked. As he walked he looked back at the building and idly wondered again why the architecture reminded him of the University of Mexico in Albuquerque. It was at that moment that something inside his mind made the decision. It wasn't sudden; it had been lurking in the back of his mind for days. He'd take a ride—the kind of ride the doctor who had lived across the street had taken; a final ride. But, he'd make his different—no booze, no pills. There would be no way to know or to guess whether or not it was suicide. He'd be cold sober, obey the speed limit and make it look good. Then, those who hated him would not know for sure whether or not his own misery had gotten to him.

Once his mind was made up and the matter settled, there was no reason to delay. He'd go home to bed, sleep for a while, wake up at twelve-thirty a.m. and go for his last drive. He didn't take the direct route home, but drove around a while looking for the place that would be best to stage his accident. He'd need to hit something so solid that even at only legal speed, he could be assured of being killed. The thought of death didn't awe him. He wasn't sure that there was another life on the other side of death, nor did he know that if it did exist it would be any better or worse than what he was living. He guessed that what he was hoping for was oblivion.

His present state of depression could be taken care of easily. He could take an "upper" and then get some rest. This would make him feel better, but to what end? He'd go back to work, work himself to a frazzle and into a deeper depression. A smile crossed his face as he thought of the words from a song sung by Fred Astaire ". . . Let's call the whole thing off . . ."

At home he found that the children were in bed and Cathy was in the master bedroom. She didn't speak to him and he kept his silence. Each knew that any conversation would lead to argument. Arguments had been the order of the day and the order of the night for weeks. They were both so tired of it that silence was to be preferred. Chuck got into his pajamas, climbed into bed and closed his eyes. Cathy, book in hand, climbed in and stayed strictly on her own side. She read for a few minutes and then turned out the light and rolled over on her side away from him. Neither said a good night. In a moment or two, both were asleep

Chuck hadn't set his alarm, and yet right on the minute he woke up. It was twelve-thirty a.m. He lay quietly for a moment until he was sure that Cathy was still asleep. The only sound other than his wife's steady breathing was the nightingale singing outside his bedroom window. Could he have gotten his hands on the bird, he'd have throttled it. He hated the sound.

Satisfied that no one else in the house was

awake, he got out of bed. Years of experience that had come with the practice of medicine and its midnight calls enabled him to dress and leave the room, and do it all silently. He walked down the hall in the dark without touching anything and turned toward the kitchen. It was through the kitchen that he'd leave the house and get to the garage and his car.

He didn't get through the kitchen. Halfway across the room, when he was about even with the middle of the kitchen table, he bumped into someone. He walked around to the other side of the table but the same thing happened again. He couldn't get through on that side either.

He whispered to himself. "What gives?"

He tried both sides of the table again but it was as though a transparent person met him in the middle of the room. Suddenly something unexpected happened. He began to get the inner sensation he'd experienced when the girl from San Francisco had been talking in the Parish Hall. Then his mind went back even further. He could see himself standing beside his grandmother, standing in a Christian and Missionary Alliance tent meeting listening to the invitation "to come forward and accept Christ." He had almost gone forward that Sunday, but even though he didn't go, he had stood in his place and had repeated the words of conversion to himself, but he had done so silently, he hadn't really said them out loud. Now he spoke louder than he had ever remembered speaking, "Forgive me my sins as I forgive . . . Oh God, Oh God."

A verse that his grandmother had taught him

came to mind, a verse found in the book of Romans, "If you confess with your mouth the Lord Jesus . . ." That was it, the part he had never done. Now he would say it.

The edge of the sink became an altar and he was on his knees sobbing. Then something strange happened to him again. He could see, coming out of his mouth, a stream of garbage and junk. It came out, went up in a constant stream and dissipated into nothing. It was as though everything that was rotten in him was being pulled out of him. When the vision was finally over, Chuck was still on his knees sobbing. But now the agony was gone and the tears flowed accompanied by a sense of relief and joy. He himself was now experiencing the experience that he had heard described. Finally he could say what he wanted to say, simply and clearly, "Jesus, you are my Savior and my Lord."

He wanted to continue praying but he needed more words. Then he remembered that he had been at a political meeting a couple of weeks previously where someone had prayed the St. Francis prayer and Chuck had been impressed. He tried to continue by praying that prayer. "Lord, make me a channel of thy peace—that where there is hatred, I may bring love—that where there is wrong, I may bring the spirit of forgiveness—that where there is error, I may bring truth . . . And Lord, I don't remember the rest of it, but I mean that part too. Amen."

He got up off his knees and went back to the bedroom. Cathy was still breathing steadily. Whatever noise he had made in the kitchen had not disturbed anyone. God must have seen to that; he'd made plenty. He undressed and got back into bed. As he lay there listening, he heard the nightingale's song again. In the last hour or two, it had changed from an annoying irritant into a beautiful melody, one that could be created only by a loving God. In a few minutes he was asleep.

PART II

RT-1 PRESENT ILLNESS: (Continued) He became possessed with ideas of his own increasing religious sensitivity and supernatural powers . . . He became increasingly involved in his grandiosity and his religious delusions and this began to affect his relationship to his medical colleagues and even in his practice . . .

16 Sept 64
MODESTO

About five o'clock Wednesday morning Chuck awoke. He found himself filled with a sense of love; love for the woman lying beside him, love for his children, love for all of God's children, love for all men. It was almost a physical sensation, as though he were wrapped in it. He lay quietly enjoying his new found peace, then as the room grew lighter, he discovered that the nightingale's song was not the only thing that had changed. Until that morning, his vision had been a real problem, correctable to normal, but a very large correction. Without his thick glasses he couldn't see across the room. That was not so any longer. By the time the room was completely filled with the rising sun, he could see the wallpaper pattern on the wall of the room far more clearly without his glasses than he ever had seen it with them.

He lay quietly on his bed to think the thing through. Finally it occurred to him that because God had given him spiritual sight to know who and what Jesus Christ was, God had given him physical sight too. It was a sign of what had happened. He lay still with his eyes re-closed until Cathy was awakened by one of the children stirring. With a disgruntled noise she got out of bed to fix breakfast for the family.

Chuck didn't move. He had a problem. How much should he say?

After some silent prayer he decided to say nothing until questions were asked. He then got up, bathed, shaved and dressed. With his glasses in his pocket, he went to breakfast. No one said anything. This was not too surprising, as he analyzed the situation. No one in the family wanted to look him in the eye. As he thought about it, he had to face the fact that none of them had wanted to look at him squarely for a long, long time. He'd have to change that.

To his surprise, he found the same thing happening during his hospital calls. No one said anything about his missing glasses.

Doctors Hospital was the third and last, so he left there for the Medical Group, drove to the parking lot and pulled into his spot. The walk from his car to the building was a pleasure; he was enjoying a quality and quantity of vision that he had never known before. He even started humming one of the choir tunes he had learned when he'd been a boy soprano in the Episcopal Church. Neither the words nor the music had crossed his mind for years.

As he entered the Medical Group building, the first doctor he saw was his opthalmologist, Jerry. Jerry was one of the few members of the Medical Group who was a friend of Chuck's. The two doctors had certain superficial qualities in common, including a mutual love for contract bridge, which they played together whenever they could squeeze in the time.

Jerry spent his life looking at eyes, and the absence of Chuck's glasses was immediately noticed.

"Where are your glasses?"

"I don't need them any more." Chuck was grinning from ear to ear.

"Don't try to tell that to a cop if you get stopped while driving without them. You're so myopic you can't see across the street unless you have them on."

"Try me."

They walked to a window where the sign on a building a long way away could be seen. The opthalmologist still had a feeling that he was getting his leg pulled. He pointed to the sign. "Read it backward if you can see it."

Chuck read the letters backward, rapidly and without any hesitation. Then he asked Jerry a question. "You're the opthalmologist, you prescribed my glasses. Why don't you put me in your chair and check my eyes?"

When the test was over, Jerry didn't believe the results. He tested them again. He got the same answer. Chuck's eyes were better than normal, particularly for distance vision. He was stumped.

"Come on, Chuck, what did you do, and don't put me on."

Because of the night's events, Chuck was free of guile, but was short on experience when it came to sharing spiritual things. As it turned out, it might have been a good thing for him to have held his peace, at least for a time. In the Gospels, Jesus healed more than one person and then told the healed man to keep his mouth shut about it. Chuck opened his.

"I'll tell you what happened. I was walking through the dark kitchen of my home last night at twelve-thirty in the morning on my way to my car. I was going to drive it into an abuttment and commit suicide. I never got through the kitchen. Jesus Christ met me there, in my kitchen, and He wouldn't let me through. He emptied me of my sins and he gave me spiritual vision. As a sign of this, He gave me physical vision too."

The opthalmologist looked at Chuck in a peculiar way and rendered a verdict that was soon to become universal. He said it in a quiet and friendly way, but he said it.

"You're crazy."

PART III

That same day, Chuck finished his rounds later than usual. By the time he got home, Cathy was already in her night gown and in bed reading. Chuck walked into the room and removed his coat and started to remove his tie. He spoke to Cathy as nicely as he knew how.

"Hi, how you doin'?"

She looked up at him without answering his question. "You win, I'll ask. Where are your glasses? You didn't have them on this morning either."

"You noticed?"

"Yes, I noticed."

"I don't need them any more."

"You've got contacts?"

"Nope." He walked close to her on her side of the bed and bent over, pointing to his eyes. "No lenses."

Then he walked over to the foot of their bed. The book she was reading had reasonably large type. "Turn your book toward me."

She did and he started reading it from the foot of the bed.

She closed the book and looked at him quizzically. "What happened?"

He told her the same story he'd told the opthalmologist, only he told it in greater detail. The result was the same, and the same remark came out, only in a less friendly manner.

"You're crazy."

"Is my new vision crazy?"

"I don't know. Maybe it is some quirk in your head."

"I've studied a lot of psychiatry, but I don't remember any name or description of a 'quirk' like that. Furthermore, I think I might have another 'quirk', a very nice one."

"Oh." There was a little edge to her voice. "What's that?"

"Well, you do what you call 'your wifely duty' and we'll both find out." He took her in his arms more gently than he ever had before.

An hour later, Cathy was exhausted and crying.

"Cathy, why are you crying? That was great."

"It was great for you, but I hate it. I hate losing control of myself like that. What happened to you?"

"Well, I think that in the past I've had a lot of guilt, and a lack of self-acceptance. I covered it over with fake macho and hard medicine. Jesus Christ has taken away the guilt and I can accept myself. I don't have to try to prove anything."

"What's that got to do with sex?"

"A great deal indeed. I'm not afraid of failure anymore, so I don't fail."

"I'm going to see a psychiatrist."

"If you want to go that route, see Dr. Hill in Stockton.

"I don't want to see him about me, I want to talk to him about you."

Chuck smiled. "If you tell him you don't enjoy normal sex, you're the one who's going to be the patient." He didn't know how wrong he was.

Cathy climbed out of bed and grabbed her night clothes. She started putting them back on. He watched her for a moment before he spoke.

"Where are you going?"

"I'm going to sleep out on the couch. You've changed so much, I don't know what you'll do next. I may wake up and find my throat slit."

"Cathy, I wouldn't hurt you for the world. There is nothing in my heart anymore but love for you, both kinds, and God's put them both there."

She fastened her bathrobe as she went through the door and she was still crying angry tears. "You can go to hell."

The next morning, Chuck went to the breakfast table still minus his glasses and still minus his irritating manner. He spoke cheerfully and kindly to his children. None of them knew how to handle it. The five children, who ranged in age from thirteen down to three, thought that their irritating and easily irritated father was in one of his rare and temporary good moods. They were sure this one wouldn't last either.

Cathy was sure of the same thing as she spoke to them. "It's all right, children," she spoke from in front of the stove, "This is your father's week to be an Eagle Scout. He will be his usual nasty self in a few days."

He wasn't. Day after day went by and the cheerfulness and kindness continued. The children were intrigued and he might have gradually worked his way through their long standing dislike of him, if it hadn't been for Cathy. She and her children had been against him for years, and she was out to see that the status didn't change. She fought like a tiger and she succeeded in what she wanted; she kept the wall up between Chuck and his children, but one other thing that she desperately desired didn't come her way. He didn't lose his temper nor did he "answer in kind."

Weeks after his conversion experience, he still hadn't changed back to "himself." He still needed no glasses. He even walked differently. The weight of the world was no longer on his shoulders; the weight now belonged to God. Chuck had given it back to God. With that weight gone, he could stand up straighter and walk confidently. Besides the change in posture, there was another change. He broke a habit he had tried to break for years, the habit of biting his nails to the quick. It would be more accurate to say that it broke itself. There was no conscious effort on his part, and along with this, the pencils he carried were no longer marred with teeth marks.

Cathy was frustrated. Her ring-in-the-nose-bedroom-slave had become both solidly masculine and at the same time very gentle. She no longer controlled the situation. She had gone to see Dr. Hill, the psychiatrist, but it had not been a bit satisfactory. Instead of agreeing with her that her husband was crazy, he had asked some questions suggesting that she might find a bit of a problem in herself. She switched psychiatrists.

With the second shrink, she held the conversations to the subject of Chuck and started building her case. This began to re-shift the leverage back to Cathy for there was a growing sense of oppression on Chuck when he was at home. At first he couldn't figure it out, but then gradually he began to see that Cathy really did think he was genuinely crazy. This put him in the position of having to prove himself sane. That is not easy to do when someone really wants to believe that you are not.

There was pressure at the church too. He talked to the Episcopal pastor, a man who was honestly delighted with the doctor's conversion, and invited Chuck to a Bible study fellowship group that met mid-week. Things in that group were soon strained. In the first place, Chuck's testimony was rather spectacular, disconcertingly so to some Episcopalians. Added to this was Chuck's problem, characteristic of many people who have been suddenly and dramatically turned around to God. He was apt to be a little suspicious of the genuineness of the Christian who hasn't had a dramatic conversion. Subconsciously and not at all deliberately, he made many in the group who had entered God's Kingdom gradually seem like second-class citizens.

Also, Chuck had a hunger for Scripture that was insatiable. He pored over it as he studied it like he had not studied anything since he'd left medical school. He didn't see why the Bible study had to stop at nine o'clock, and he said so. Why not go on until midnight? This caused a certain uneasiness.

None of this was doing anything good to his relationship with the Medical Group. His few friends in the Group were somewhat enstranged by the force and insistence of his testimony. They were a little upset by the complete change in his personality. Anyone who would have picked him for a friend before his conversion, would not be attracted by the post-conversion model. As far as his enemies were concerned, and there were several of those, they were happy to pass the word that, "Old Chuck has flipped."

Some of his wealthier patients disappeared also. They didn't care to "have a word of prayer" about their child's illness. They just switched doctors. This should have led to a confrontation, but there was a mitigating factor that kept things from coming to a head. The factor that delayed the coming confrontation was the quality of Chuck's medicine. It had been good, but now it was better, and now he gave credit to God when he found something that another doctor had missed. The old conceit was gone. Most of the doctors would have liked to have it back in place of the newly found "religion." But, what do you do with a physician who finds something that saves your patient pain and suffering, and sometimes saves the patient's life? That kind of doctor is not easy to fire.

In the end, Chuck went too far. He was uninstructed, wildly enthusiastic, and he wouldn't stop talking about Christ. Heat was generated in certain quarters, and about four months after his conversion, Chuck got a phone call from the doctor who was President of the Medical Group. The call was expected; Chuck knew it was coming.

"Chuck, this is Bert."

"Yes, sir. What may I do for you?" He was surprised at the evenness of his voice and at how casually he was taking this call.

"I might as well come right to the point." This was nothing new, he always did. His voice was harsh and cold. "We like the quality of your medicine, but we're a little disappointed in its shrinking quantity. The practice of medicine is a full time job, you know that, and other interests crowd in, and they get in the way."

Chuck decided to state his case and let the chips fall. "Sometimes 'interests' as you put it, get themselves pushed in. Nothing has happened to me that I've asked for. God has intervened in my life uninvited, and I'm happy about it regardless of the cost. I'm at peace with my Creator. Less important, but none the less invaluable, I'm more at peace with myself, and good things have happened. I can see without glasses, I can stand up straight without even trying, and some other problems have cleared up. What is more important from your point of view, I'm learning things about medicine that are not taught in med school. I believe that God is teaching me."

He had wasted his breath. "Chuck, you can blame God if you want to, but I've seen this sort of thing before. You're headed for a breakdown and you're going to have it if you don't turn yourself around and get your mind off religion.

"Also to be considered are the interests of the Medical Group which are two-fold. First, we've some men in the Group we'd like to keep who say they are getting to the place where they'll leave if you don't, or at least if you don't shut up about religion. Now, I'm going to help you channel this. The county medical society has been asked to send a doctor to join a group of clergymen, psychologists and psychiatrists who are going to be a committee called 'Religion and Medicine.' We're trying to get more cooperation and help from the clergy, particularly with terminal cases. I will recommend to the society that they choose you for that committee. That way you can talk about your beliefs in an appropriate place and at an appropriate time.

"Second, Chuck, as you well know you've slowed way down. You're taking far more time per patient, and your practice is picking up an unusual number of dead beats. People who do not pay their bills are of no help to the Medical Group, they should be going to a clinic."

"I treat anyone who needs help." On this point Chuck felt he was on firmer ground. "I think there's an oath somewhere to that effect."

The voice got icy. "Yes, of course. Well, let's put it this way. As long as that oath is so important to you it would seem to be in the best interests of the Medical Group if we reduced your salary by five thousand a year beginning next month and for as long as you decide to stay with us."

In other words, find another job.

"That will be fair," Chuck responded. "I'll take that. I shall also try to be a little more discreet."

There was a flat finality in Bert's voice. "That will be much appreciated." He hung up.

Chuck had to move his family. He could no longer afford a thirty-six hundred square foot home on the edge of the creek with its three car garage. They sold the house and moved into a more modest tract, not small houses, theirs had twenty-seven hundred square feet, but it was far less prestigious. The children went to different schools and were with children who were not in the financial brackets they'd grown used to. Also, Cathy had problems. She didn't have as much time for the racquet club and she had to do more of her own housework. She was no longer angry, she was furious.

CHAPTER FOUR

PART I

RT-1 PRESENT ILLNESS: (Continued) On Rorschach, he (Sweigard) saw nothing but penises and vaginas on every card and he demonstrated a constant desperate groping for relatedness of which he ambivalently was afraid.

(Approximately six weeks after entering Langley Porter.)

16 Oct 65
SAN FRANCISCO

Chuck knew now that when he had taken his Rorschach test he had blown it. He had tried to be clever, but he'd been in over his head. The psychiatric studies in med school had been quite extensive, but many years had gone by, and his memory had faded. In trying to figure out what it was that the psychiatrist wanted to hear, he did a very bad job in deed. He knew the man had strong Freudian tendencies and would be heavy on the sex aspect of the test, but Chuck's half-forgotten psychiatry got him into a hole.

Then he made another mistake. Seeing that he was getting nowhere with the psychiatrist, he changed horses in the middle of the stream and tried to talk about where he really was and what had really happened. The combination was a mess. As he thought back on that experience, he had to admit to himself that he'd given to the psychiatrists grounds to cause him a lot of further trouble.

The young doctor at Langley Porter who was in charge of Chuck's case had a lot to go on, and he was using it. Every session was a battle as they sat across the table from each other and fought. It was not a fair fight. All the ammunition was on the side of the psychiatrist. What ammunition Chuck did have, he used poorly. His mental facilities were muddied up with drugs and the drugs also made recollection difficult. It took a lot of effort to try to remember what he had learned in school. Also, the drugs had an effect on his will. They made it harder and harder to fight. It would have been so easy to give in, disavow his conversion and his subsequent experiences, admit that it was all a figment of his imagination, and then begin to "get well" and go home. There was a fierce desire to take that easy route, but he would not, he could not, bring himself to say that his confrontation with the risen Christ had been insanity.

This was a Saturday. There would be no sessions today, and the patients thought capable would be permitted to go for a walk. He was among those who would be allowed to leave. There was no fear on the part of the staff as to the possibility of his running away. He couldn't run. He could hardly walk. The drugs had caught up to him and he moved with the awkwardness that characterized all patients.

His manner of walk made escape impossible for another reason. Not only did he have to move slowly, but the characteristics of his walk were known to every cop in San Francisco and any who saw him too far from the hospital would pick him up and take him back. Besides all that, what would he do if he got away? His medical license had been suspended when he had been declared insane. What would he do for a living? Where would he get money?

These factors were important but there was one overriding objection to his running. He was at Langley Porter for a purpose. He was going through what he was going through for a reason, Jesus Christ was sovereign. He had read that statement in Matthew during his devotions. They weren't private devotions, there were twelve men in the ward, but they were semi-private, nobody paid any attention to him as he read, and as he finished the Gospel that verse had spoken to his heart. "All authority in heaven and on earth has been given to me . . ." That meant power over Langley Porter too, and Chuck would walk out of the hospital the day that Jesus opened the door, not a day early, not a day late. He would have to stay and fight for his sanity until he had learned whatever it was God wanted him to learn.

One of the attendants poked his head into the ward. "It's time for your walk, any of you who want to are free to go."

They made a pathetic sight as they exited the building on to Parnassus Ave., a half-dozen men with their shuffling awkward walk, as though they had severe lumbago and a light case of St. Vitus Dance. Anyone in the neighborhood who saw them knew who and what they were. The humiliation was not as hard to take as continuous confinement; Chuck would go through almost anything to get out of the place if only for an hour.

They shuffled east toward Stanyan where there was a food store, a place where they could get things to eat that weren't on the hospital menu. As they walked, Chuck could see a few of the top seats in the top rows of the east end of Kezar Stadium. He wondered idly if the Forty-niners were playing there the next afternoon. He had read the schedule but he couldn't remember. There were lots of things he couldn't remember. If the team did play there the following day, there'd be no parking place for miles in any direction, there would be cars everywhere. Worse, the cheers of the crowd would be heard in the ward. It was one more frustrating factor in his life, that though he could hear he could not see. When the team played at home there was no local TV. Even that was losing its appeal. The drugs were affecting his sight, and the excellent vision God had given him was weakening. TV was harder and harder to watch. And now he needed a magnifying glass when he read.

The walk down Parnassus was slow but not painful, it was the steep walk back up that was agony. In the crazy world in which Chuck lived, everything that went down had to come up. They reached the doughnut shop, had their snack and then began their crawl back up the hill. Chuck finally made it and sat down gratefully on his bed. He would have given anything he had ever owned for the privilege of lying down, but that was strictly forbidden. No matter how painful the process, patients stayed up during the day and lay down only during the night. If a patient was uncooperative, about this and other things too, the psychiatrist could always recommend "shock therapy" after which the patient cooperated no matter what. Chuck had seen enough of that horror in med school, and he would avoid it if he could.

He pulled out his Bible and his magnifying glass and began to read and to pray. He had to get ready for next week's "consultations" with the psychiatrist, and Bible reading and prayer were the best help he could find. There was no fellowship. He had asked to see a minister of the Gospel. They had picked one for him from the hospital's approved list. The minister had come as requested and had talked to Chuck. He was an assistant minister who was attached to the staff of Bishop Pike's Church. After three minutes of conversation, Chuck felt sure the man was a homosexual and there would be no fellowship in Christ. They spent the hour in desultory conversation. Chuck never asked to have him back.

The next Monday there was a change in schedule. The expected consultation did not occur. In place of consultations there was an assembly. They were to hear from a special guest, someone who was giving her time to help the sick. At about ten in the morning, the patients shuffled into a large room which served as an auditorium and there they took their seats. One of the young doctors got up and made a little speech.

"We are very privileged to have an honored guest today. As you know, we all must pattern ourselves after someone, and it is helpful when a great human being allows us to share in their personality, their thinking and their talent. We have such a person this morning, someone who is truly a friend to us all. May I present Joan Baez."

There was scattered applause, mostly from the doctors. Joan took a chair at the front of the room and began to play her guitar. Then she sang. She sang about loving our fellowman, about loving life, and about keeping our planet green.

When it was over Chuck shuffled out with the rest and went back to his bed. He searched in vain among his personal belongings for his Bible. It was gone. He went to the nurse's station. It was the same nurse who had given him his first shot. Her face hardened at the sight of him. He was rather glad to see that she really didn't like her job and had to force herself to do it. She spoke first.

"What may I do for you, Dr. Sweigard?"

"I can't find my Bible, did someone take it?"

"Yes, I did. Your doctor told me to. He said it was one of the things that was making you sick. I'm sorry."

Chuck shuffled back to his bed.

PART II

RT-1 PRESENT ILLNESS: (Continued) The severity of his mental illness became more pronounced during the recent week or two and at the present time, quite florid. He now believes that he is actually Jesus Christ returned to earth to perform His God-like mission and to save mankind but he feels there will be an enormous holocaust before the kingdom of God is established . . .

30 July 65
MODESTO
(Before Commitment)

It was a Friday afternoon and Chuck was in the backyard of their home on Edgebrook Drive. His backyard was going to look like a jungle if he didn't work on it. Now that Cathy had no help in the house, and had not had for several months, he didn't feel at liberty to hire a gardener. His practice had slowed down to the place where he could take an afternoon off once a week and work on the yard. He rather enjoyed it and worked hard and fast in spite of the heat.

He was at home alone. Cathy had gone shopping and taken the youngest ones with her. She never let him have any time with them alone if she could help it. She was afraid Chuck might talk to them about the Lord, or try to pray with them. She wanted to keep her platoon solidly in place, ready to repel any attempted intrusion from Chuck. Her children were going to be "protected" from any of his crazy ideas. Although she worried about all the children, she worried less about the older ones. She had spent time conditioning them against anything their father might say, and they were less impressionable. Also, they were picking up friends and lives of their own. They spent their afternoons at the public swimming pool. She would have far rather had them swimming at the racquet club, but they couldn't afford membership. That angered her every time she thought about it, no matter how many times she thought about it.

Chuck was absorbed in his gardening and his praying. He jumped when suddenly he realized he was not alone. The stranger spoke immediately.

"I didn't mean to startle you. You looked busy and like you were concentrating on something and I didn't want to interrupt."

"That's all right. What may I do for you?"

The man handed him a card that showed he was a home delivery milk man for one of the local dairies. "My name is Jim, and I'm trying to build up my milk route. A couple of your neighbors are customers of mine and I thought I'd like to talk to you. I think your neighbors will recommend me."

Chuck put the man's card in his pocket as he spoke. "It would be all right with me, but on this subject my wife Cathy has the last word. I'm afraid you'll have to talk to her." In those days Chuck gave his "testimony" to anything that moved, and he begin looking for an opening to bring the conversation around to the subject of Jesus Christ. "Do you live around here, Jim?"

"No, I live near the dairy. If you don't mind my asking, what's your line of work?"

"I'm an M.D., a pediatrician."

"It's strange to see one of those doing his own yard work."

This provided the opening for which Chuck was waiting. "I enjoy it, I need the exercise, and I'm not as well off as most doctors."

"Oh?"

"Yes, you see, I've had an encounter with the living Jesus Christ, and my interest in telling others about it has somewhat diminished my medical practice."

"Praise God!" Jim practically exploded. "Tell me about it."

Chuck did. The two men stood in the broiling sun, one talking and one listening, both oblivious to the heat. When Chuck was through, Jim exploded again. "Praise God, praise God!"

For Chuck this was a new experience. It was the first time since his conversion that he had given his account to someone who believed it wholeheartedly, and went along with him and his story without question or mental reservations. It was a precious experience for him and it gave him a very warm feeling toward Jim. He asked Jim the obvious question.

"I gather, you're a believer."

"Oh," said Jim, "more than that. I've had the second blessing. I have received the Baptism of the Holy Spirit."

"I've heard of a group that talks that way."

"Yes, we're called Pentecostals." Jim proceeded to give Chuck his testimony and Chuck listened with interest. When the personal testimony was complete, Jim took a small tract out of his pocket and gave it to Chuck. "Could you come to our church Sunday?"

"No, I'm on call Sunday and I can't leave the phone."

"How about the next week? Sunday night at seven on August eighth we're having a Holy Spirit Baptism service, could you come to that?"

Chuck was intrigued. "I'll try."

Jim was a tall, lean man with an honest and wholesome face, a face that was divided at the moment by a large grin. He'd found a genuine Holy Spirit Baptism candidate. "Doctor, you read that tract, and you look up all those Bible verses and then you come to our service. The address of our church is stamped on the back of the tract. Will you come?"

Chuck smiled. "As I said, I'll try."

Jim left, too happy to remember to ask Chuck when he would be able to talk to Cathy about the milk delivery.

PART III

8 Aug 65
MODESTO

Chuck walked into the Pentecostal church at seven-fifteen. That meant he was fifteen minutes late. He was late because he had delayed his departure from home until he had a chance to leave in such a way that there would be no questions. If someone were to ask him where he was going, he wouldn't want to say, to a Pentecostal Church, nor would he want to lie. He waited until the moment arrived when everyone in the house was busy with their own thing, then he took off.

The church had folding chairs placed in traditional rows. There was a raised platform at the front of the room and an upright piano against the wall on the song leader's left. He was leading the congregation in the singing of a song that Chuck had never heard. It was rather "jazzy" and was not something sung in an Episcopal Church. The singing was lusty. Chuck noticed that some people had their heads back and their eyes closed. They knew the song well, and needed to look at neither words nor music.

As soon as the song finished, there were cries of "Amen" and "Praise God" and "Be with us Holy Spirit."

The song leader, a good-looking, dark-haired young man wearing a rather expensive suit, had seen Chuck enter, and he had nodded to Jim. Apparently they had been expecting Jim's new found friend. The milk man was so tall that he could see over the rest of the crowd. After the song leader nodded to him he turned and gave Chuck a happy smile and a nod.

After the song, as the murmur died down, the song leader lifted both his hands above his head, fingers out-stretched and said, "Let's all praise God!"

Something close to bedlam ensued and Chuck watched with interest. He heard some sounds coming out of two people a couple of rows in front of him and presumed that that was "speaking in tongues." Almost everyone had their hands in the air, shouting and praising and saying Hallelujah. He felt no desire to join in, but to his surprise he wasn't offended. When that session had ended, the songleader told the congregation that Brother Jim had had the pleasure of meeting someone a couple of weeks previously, "Someone who had had an encounter with God, a man who has talked with the Holy Spirit in an encounter with Jesus. And now we're going to ask that man to come forward and share his experience with us at this time. Doctor, won't you please come forward."

Chuck was taken by surprise, but felt no resentment and went forward to the platform. He began his story, and as he went along, the crowd went with him. There were cries of "Isn't Jesus Wonderful" and "Praise God."

Except for Jim, Chuck had never told his story to anyone who unreservedly believed it, and now telling it to a group of people, all of whom believed it, all of it, gave him an emotional lift.

When he was through, the pastor of the Pentecostal Church began his sermon. It was well-paced and the crowd was raised to a fever pitch. When the invitation to receive the baptism was given, to the delight of all present, Chuck went forward. He knelt and hands were laid on him. The pastor prayed fervently that Brother Chuck would receive the Baptism of the Holy Spirit.

Chuck drove home in a state of near ecstasy. The ecstasy ended when he got home to Cathy. She was waiting for him in her usual evening position, in her night clothes and in bed with a book.

"Where have you been?"

Not anticipating the explosion that was coming, Chuck answered innocently enough. "I went to a Pentecostal meeting and gave my testimony. After the service I went forward and they laid hands on me and prayed that I'd receive the Baptism of the Holy Spirit."

From the size of the eruption that followed that announcement, he might just as well have said that he had just blown up the city hall. Cathy's fury knew no bounds, and there was reason for it. As long as Chuck was the only person who believed Chuck, she had reason to believe that the "crazy dream," as she called it, would fade. He'd come back to his senses, back to his full-time practice of medicine with its attendant income. All this was now threatened. If he had found a group of people as crazy as he was, or crazier, he'd get the support that he needed to go on believing his stupid hallucination.

When she paused for a breath to go on upbraiding him, he had a chance to get in a word or two. "Why are you so angry? I haven't hurt anyone."

"You've hurt me, stupid. Do you think I want to be known as the wife of a doctor who is so crazy he attends a Pentecostal Church and speaks there? You've hurt your children too. You know how cruel kids can be. What are your children going to say when they are teased at school, and teased they will be. This God-forsaken place is still a small town, and your nutty behavior is going to be known all over it. I'm not even going to want to go to the grocery store. Supposing I bump into one of those nuts and they speak to me?"

She hurled her book across the room. "Chuck, how could you do this to us, how could you?"

"I haven't done anything wrong. I feel more freedom, more love—"

"Oh, shut up. We're not sharing any bed tonight. You can have the couch. Get out of here."

Chuck quietly reached in the closet for his pajamas and bathrobe. He took them and left. As he did so, he heard her lock the bedroom door behind him. That didn't worry him particularly. Cathy wanted to be a doctor's wife, she still dreamed of returning to social glory and to the ranks of the economically privileged. He was her only possible ticket back to the upper echelons. She would try to change him and try as hard as she dared, but she wouldn't shut him out for long. So, while she still

didn't enjoy sex as she should, she was smart
enough to work at it. It was the only gun left in her
arsenal. The door might be locked Sunday night,
but it would be unlocked on Monday.

PART IV

24 Aug 65
MODESTO

The room was dark when Chuck awoke. The
first signs of dawn were still an hour or two away.
The strange thing was that he was seeing something
he never expected to see. When he opened his eyes,
he had the view from the cross, the view of the faces
looking up at the dying Jesus. The whole crowd was
there, the weeping women, the forlorn disciples and
the jeering members of the Sanhedren.

The faces of the crowd dimmed and then blended with another scene. The new scene gradually
took over. Chuck was looking at an attack on a
small city, the attack was being made by Genghis
Khan. He saw the bloodshed and the violent
deaths. Slowly that scene faded only to be followed
by another; the troops on the plains of Marathos.
One by one the scenes blended, following one another, with each in its turn becoming clear before
blending again into the next scene. He saw the pha-
lanx of Alexander, their closed ranks and closed
files, their joined shields and their overlapping
spears. They gave way to the legions of Rome, and

these in turn to the Crusades, the terrible battles between Catholic and Turk. History unrolled its bloody and terrible story of conflict, agony and death.

The last part of the vision was the worst. Chuck could see a concentration camp in Hitler's Germany, and then as though he had a zoom lense he moved forward to one building, and then to the inside of that building. He had never seen anything like that, he had never seen any pictures like that, he did not know that one man could do such things to another.

Finally the vision ended. He lay in bed quietly weeping. Then he began to pray.

"Lord, now I know why you died, you died to pay for all this, to put an end to all this, to bring in your kingdom of love and peace. God, make me one of your instruments."

Then he began sobbing uncontrollably and in so doing, he woke Cathy.

"Now, what is the matter with you?"

"I've just had the view that Christ had from the cross."

"You are totally, completely and utterly nuts. Shut up and go back to sleep." She rolled over on to her side. Her back was toward him.

"Would you get me a drink of water please?" Chuck asked.

"Why don't you get it yourself?"

"I can't move." He couldn't. All strength was drained out of him. He thought of the Old Testament quote in the 22nd Psalm. "I am poured out like water, and all my bones are out of joint . . . "

Cathy got out of bed, slid her feet into her slippers and went into the bathroom for water. She handed the glass to him, but he couldn't raise his hand. He couldn't raise his head either. She put one hand behind it, raised it and put the glass to his lips. He drank thirstily, all of it.

"Do you want some more?"

"No, thank you."

"You really can't move, can you?"

"No."

She returned the glass to its place in the bathroom and went to the phone. The first call was to Dr. Hill in Stockton. His answering service said that he was out of town until Monday. Then she tried her own psychiatrist in Modesto. He too was unavailable. The third call was to the pastor of a church, a pastor whom she had met at the racquet club. He was a fairly young man who had played a decent game of tennis and he and Cathy had gotten acquainted. He was the one who had approached her. He had heard about Chuck's conversion and was interested in the doctor. The pastor had pleaded Chuck's case with Cathy, trying to help the situation. That is, he tried to help until the Pentecostal experience. The man was the pastor of a Fundamentalist church and they were set against Pentecostalism. As soon as Chuck's friendship with Pentecostals had been reported to him, he had been upset and had given Cathy a very sympathetic ear. He agreed with her that her husband had taken a bad step. He would try to help him.

He did try, but his conversation with Chuck the following day had been fruitless. However, it had not been an unfriendly conversation. The minister thought of Chuck as a new convert who had been terribly misled. To him the Baptism of the Holy Spirit was a one time, first century affair and was not to be repeated in the twentieth century. He had called Cathy and told her so, and so from Cathy's point of view, the pastor seemed like a good man to approach with the present problem. His phone rang for a while before it was answered.

A sleepy voice said, "Hello."

"This is Cathy Sweigard."

"Yes, ma'am, what may I do for you?"

"I'm sorry to disturb you at this hour, but my husband has really flipped out. He thinks he is Jesus on the cross and he's catatonic."

Neither assertion was true, Chuck had said that he had seen through the eyes of Jesus. He had not said that He'd confused his personality. Secondly, he was not catatonic. People who are catatonic are stiff as boards, and can't talk. Chuck could talk and was was no more rigid than a lump of Jello.

"Mrs. Sweigard, have you called a psychiatrist?"

"Two of them, his and mine. Neither is available, can you help?"

There was a moment's pause before the pastor answered. This situation could be a little over his head. He'd need counsel. "I'm very sorry indeed about what has happened, Mrs. Sweigard, but I'm not surprised. Pentecostalism leads to this sort of thing, but let me see what I can do. I'll call one of my elders who is an M.D. and have him come with me. We'll be right over."

Cathy said her thank you and hung up. Then she got dressed and went to the front door to let them in when they came. They arrived in about fifteen minutes, and she ushered them into the bedroom. The Fundamentalist doctor had brought his bag, and he took out the paraphernalia needed to take Chuck's blood pressure and pulse. Both were normal. Then he started asking questions.

As Chuck talked about what he had seen and what he'd been through, things got worse and worse. It was painfully apparent that no one believed him, they obviously placed him with the "loonies." He was in a box. If he kept silent, he would seem uncooperative. If he told them a plausible story, he'd be lying. If he stuck to the truth, he'd sound crazy. He stuck to the truth. He was right; he sounded crazy.

After he finished his story, the two men and Cathy went into the other room and talked. At that moment, the nightingale whose song was now familiar and a very beautiful, opened up and started singing. It was a comfort, and Chuck remembered his prayer, the one in which he had asked for God's perfect will for his life. If this was to be a part of it, it was to be accepted.

"Lord," Chuck said prayerfully, "I think that they're about to take me to an insane asylum."

He thought he heard an audible answer, "Yes."

He heard someone dialing the phone. He presumed it was the doctor and that he was calling an ambulance. The ambulance didn't come promptly. The case was not that kind of an emergency. Also, the personnel and equipment were apt to be different when an out of town trip was involved. It took time to get things together, and so it was full daylight when the big Cadillac backed into the Sweigard driveway. Its paint job hardly made it inconspicuous. Understandably, a few of the neighbors gathered around. They were not informed that Dr. Sweigard had completely flipped his lid and that he was being taken to the State Hospital in Stockton. But Chuck knew that the truth would come out anyway; they couldn't keep it quiet for long. All this did not form the happiest set of circumstances that Chuck had ever known, but he was not troubled. He was in a state of euphoria.

In a way, it was strange that his vision would give him a sense of well-being, but it had. It was true that there had been terrible scenes in it, and yet there had been a sense of finality about the whole matter. It was as though things had already come to an end. Chuck knew now, in an experiential way, that Jesus Christ had won the battle. Time was running its dreadful course down to its catastrophic end, but more important, the end heralded the beginning, the beginning of a new and glorious world. The Lord was in control. All time, and all times, were in His hands.

Propped up in his place in the ambulance, Chuck could see well enough as they drove west on McHenry toward the freeway. They drove through air that was not yet fouled, and this in spite of the heavy flow of early morning traffic. He looked out the window at the trees, the flowers, and he took notice of the brilliant sky above him. They all combined to form an insight into the creative hand of the Lord. The lines of Wade Robinson's hymn came to mind:

Heaven above is softer blue,
Earth around is sweeter green!
Something lives in ev'ry hue
Christ-less eyes have never seen:

He began to pray for the ambulance driver, for the assistant driver, and for passing motorists.

The ambulance turned north up 99 and headed toward Stockton. The 4-story hospital's rambling administration building had a sign over the corner door that said, INFORMATION. Chuck smiled as he read it, information about what? The only information of lasting and intrinsic value was information that led to the knowledge of God.

The ambulance turned south around the administration building and went far enough to reach a break in the parkway that divided the street, and then made a U turn and headed into the semicircular drive in front of the building marked AD-MITTANCE.

The driver pulled under the portico in front of the building so as to put Chuck in the shade. The day was getting warm and the Cadillac's air condition had been running. Chuck waited while the driver went inside to announce their arrival. As he waited he saw an elderly black man cross the street a hundred feet away. The man would have been six feet five if he'd stood up straight, but he was stooped, and with his dark brown shirt and dark brown pants he seemed all of one color. He looked like a dejected human question mark, and Chuck started to pray for him.

The driver returned and the two attendants took Chuck out of their vehicle and rolled his stretcher into the building. There was a lot of scurrying around going on inside. Chuck hadn't realized how people get upset when a doctor was admitted while in Chuck's alleged condition. Doctors were gods, and they weren't supposed to go crazy. This gave rise to a lot of pitying. Chuck felt as though he were a run-over dog.

The ambulance driver went to out to park their machine, and the younger man sat down on a chair beside the stretcher. Chuck prayed, "Lord if you want me to talk to that young man, make a way."

The prayer was hardly out of his mouth before he felt strength come back into his arms. He felt relieved and mystified. He could move his hands and arms. The young man for who he had prayed spoke to him.

"Can you loan me a pencil?"

Chuck didn't know why he knew he had a pencil, he just knew that he had one.

"Certainly."

He reached into his coat pocket. It was the first time he had moved his hands since his vision. The coat was one he rarely wore. It had been put around him when they had taken him out of his house.

There was a wooden pencil in an inside pocket. Not a usual place for it in Chuck's coats, and Chuck hadn't known it was there until it was time to take it out.

With the pencil in hand, the assistant went for paper: He found some, returned to his seat and began to draw. He drew four pictures, and Chuck could see them. They reflected a disturbance in the young man's soul. The fourth picture was of a man who had a scar on his face. Chuck suddenly knew what to say.

"That man whose picture you just drew, the face with the scar on it. That man lives in San Francisco, and he had caused you a lot of trouble."

Obviously startled, the ambulance attendant sat stock still and looked at Chuck. "How did you know that?"

"God told me."

The young man shook his head unbelievingly.

Chuck pointed to one of the other pictures. It was a drawing of three incompleted arches. None of the three reached all the way from side to side, but stopped short of their obvious destinations.

"Your arches aren't completed because you can't see across into eternity. There is an arch that goes all the way, that spans the worlds. It reaches from you and your world to eternity. The name of that bridge is Jesus."

The young man sat and stared at the picture in his hand and continued to move his head from side to side silently.

CHAPTER FIVE

PART I

*THE LANGLEY PORTER NEUROPSYCHI-
ATRIC INSTITUTE*

DISCHARGE SUMMARY

Page 2   *SWEIGARD, Charles B., Jr.*
                   LPNI No. 6927

*PRESENT ILLNESS: (Continued) . . . He was
preoccupied with religion and his part in the Messian-
ic era that was forthcoming. At the urging of a minister friend and a physician the patient was taken to
Stockton County State Hospital where he was committed and subsequently transferred to Langley
Porter.*

24 Aug 64 (Continued)
STOCKTON

    An hour went by before the psychiatrist arrived.
When he did arrive, he came in a wheelchair. Chuck

took one look at him and diagnosed him correctly. Amyatrophic lateral sclerosis, terminal; the man was dying.

The psychiatrist hadn't asked many questions before Chuck realized that quick diagnosis had gone both ways. Chuck's case was closed before the questions started. The "Shrink" had a "pigeonhole mind bend." That is, he had predetermined the case, and one way or another, answers to questions that would fit his diagnosis would be found. Any answer that didn't fit into the pigeon hole would be ignored.

Suddenly things cleared, and Chuck got the picture. He remembered the psychiatrist in Modesto with whom he had had a run-in. That doctor and the one in the wheelchair would now be colleagues. Such a relationship could provide input unfavorable to Chuck. Also, there was the weight of the opinion of the Fundamentalist minister, the friend of Cathy's. The young minister had driven to Stockton, following the ambulance, and he had had an hour with the doctor before the doctor got to Chuck. That would mean that everything that Cathy could conjure up, everything that would show Chuck in a bad light, would have already gone from Cathy to the minister to the psychiatrist.

He did not hold this against Cathy. He had no way of knowing why the grace of God had fallen on him and not on her. Had things been reversed, he would have felt about her as she felt about him.

After about twenty minutes of questioning by the psychiatrist, Chuck had a pretty good idea of how he was going to be diagnosed. He was going to be labeled Schizophrenic Reaction, Paranoid Type. That was serious.

The admitting procedure took two hours. Before it was finished, the ambulance drivers had transferred him to a hospital gurney and left to go back to Modesto. The young minister was gone. There was now no connection between where Chuck was and where he had been. This was soon symbolized in a dramatic and terrifying way, for when the psychiatrist was through with the admitting examination, Chuck was wheeled through the doors that separated the world of the sane from the world of the insane. As soon as he was rolled through, the doors closed behind him. They were made of heavy metal and they banged and reverberated. He knew now where the word "slammer" came from.

Once inside, his strength began to return. In a couple of minutes he felt strength all the way down to his toes, and he knew that when he put his feet on the floor, he'd walk normally. That wasn't the only thing that changed. Up to that moment, calm and peacefulness had been his, complete peacefulness, but now it ended and the struggle began. Half of his mind said, "God's in charge, everything is all right." The other half of his mind said, "I'm sane, get me out of here." It was the beginning of a debilitating inner tension that was continued off and on for many months, for the flesh and the spirit were at war.

PART II

*30 Aug 65 RT-1 COURSE & TREATMENT (con-
tinued) . . . He sees omens and portents in every
movement, every gesticulation, every name, and every
initial. For example, his initials are C.B.S., which he
mistakenly and omnipotently interprets as Godlike
coincidence and feels that he is just like Columbia
Broadcasting System (CBS) and he has an all-seeing
eye, etc.*

30 Aug 65
STOCKTON

This was Chuck's seventh day at the Stockton
State Hospital. He had taken tests, answered questions, drawn pictures, and he had not done well. He
found himself in the same box that he had been in
when he had first had his vision. The choices were
still the same. If he told a plausible story, he was lying, if he was silent he was uncooperative, if he told
the truth he sounded crazy.

To all this, another dimension was added. He
knew enough about psychiatry to know what was
going on. Even though his medical school in Phila-
delphia had a reputation for emphasizing that
aspect of medicine, they didn't turn every doctor
into a psychiatrist, and Chuck couldn't compete
with a full time psychiatrist in the man's own field.
This meant that in trying to find answers that he
thought the doctor wanted to hear, he found an-

swers that confused the issues and made matters worse.

The respites of Saturday and Sunday were over. Monday the thirtieth began as the preceding week days had begun. The psychiatrist rolled himself into Chuck's room with his clipboard on his lap. He wanted to get his report written, he knew the judge would be at the hospital the following day. The judge would hear Chuck's case along with some others, others that might be delayed a day or two without import, but Chuck's case was pressing. His had to be adjudicated very soon. It was not wise to hold someone for more than seven days without a hearing. There could be legal complications. This would be his final conversation with Chuck.

He and Chuck said good mornings to each other and then the doctor asked a question that went off like a bomb. What did Chuck think about his future in medicine? This turned on a light, but too late. Chuck had been discussing the matter with a couple of his fellow patients. They were men to whom Chuck had tried to reach out and help. They had involved him in conversations about himself and had asked him questions they had been fed by the psychiatrist. To them Chuck had talked of his hopes of mixing preaching with the practice of medicine as soon as he got out of the institution. He told them that he had reached a point where healing bodies was not enough. He wanted to heal both body and soul, and certainly, it was more important to get men rightly related to God, more important even than keeping them well. All this information, all his conversations had been related to the psychiatrist and Chuck's answers could now be used by the doctor to fit into whatever case he wanted to make.

Once more, Chuck was in no position to lie. "I hope to mix medicine with some form of the ministry. The tests I took in college indicated that I could be a doctor or a lawyer or a minister. Maybe I'll be able to mix two of them."

"Can you imagine yourself preaching on TV?"

Chuck could imagine almost anything. "I suppose I can."

"Probably CBS?"

"Maybe."

"You've got the same initials, you know, C.B.S."

Chuck nodded. "True."

The doctor was the one who said it, but in his report he failed to give himself credit.

PART III

STOCKTON

Chuck was in a courtroom. It didn't look like a courtroom. There was no armed marshal. In place of a marshal there were two white-coated attendants. They were to take Chuck to Langley Porter when the hearing was over. In this situation, there was no attorney for the defense. The plaintiff could not read the charges. There were other differences as well. There was no "bench," just an ordinary table. The judge sat on an ordinary wooden chair and Chuck sat on one across the table from him.

Not only did it not look like a court, it didn't sound like a court. The room was silent. The judge was reading. This innocuous appearance was deceiving, for from this court could issue sentences more devastating than sentences handed out all day long in many a criminal court. This was a sanity hearing, and in 1965, the rules that protected the criminal did not always protect the patient, be he sane or insane.

The judge was a well-meaning man. He had some knowledge of mental illness, which is why he had been assigned these hearings, but he was at the mercy of the doctors. The man across from him didn't look insane, but the diagnostic impression said, "Schizophrenic Reaction—Paranoid type."

As the judge read, Chuck sat and quietly studied him and prayed. There was a battle going on in his own mind. Part of him wanted to protest to the judge, but he had some idea of the futility of that course of action. Doubtless every "Schiz" who came through the court during a period of temporary sanity argued his own case persuasively. Anything Chuck said on his own behalf would fall on preconditioned ears.

Also, there was a spiritual test in this matter. Did he, Chuck Sweigard, really believe in the sovereignty of God? If he did, on what grounds could he argue an unarguable position? Slowly he brought himself around to where, by God's grace, he could pray Christ's prayer. He prayed it silently, "Nevertheless, not my will but thy will be done."

The judge looked up at Chuck again. Then he looked back at the papers in front of him. No matter how the patient looked or acted, he had to be insane. Why would one doctor lock up another? He gave his verdict.

"This patient, Charles B. Sweigard Jr., is declared mentally incompetent and is hereby committed to the Langley Porter Neuropsychiatric Institute in San Francisco for further treatment."

With that statement, Chuck Sweigard became a ward of the State of California and subject to the ministrations of its doctors. He rose from his chair and with an attendant on each side, walked out of the court and the building, to get into the state car that would take him to San Francisco. For a man in his position, there was an incredible amount of peace in his soul.

PART IV

RT-1 PRESENT ILLNESS: (Continued) . . . He actually feels himself suspended between relatedness and nothingness, between masculinity and femininity, between life and death, etc.

18 Oct 65
SAN FRANCISCO

The group session consisted of a half a dozen patients, some relatives of some of the patients, and a psychiatrist. Chuck didn't have anyone with him at this Monday morning session, he was there alone. That would change with the session that would take place Friday afternoon. Cathy would be coming to sit in on that session and then to take him home. It was to be his first weekend away from the hospital. The promise of getting out of the place, if only for the weekend, made the thought of Cathy at the session bearable. It was going to be bad. His present state was confirmation to her that she was right, the husband she'd be taking home was crazy. The State agreed with her.

There were other aspects of going home that were not too pleasing. His present physical condition, his lack of coordination, and his awkward way of walking made him repulsive. He hated the idea of being seen by his children in his present condition, but he hated even more the idea of spending the weekend in the hospital.

When he took his seat at the Monday morning session he felt defeated and hopeless, but something happened during the subsequent conversations that proved to be a turning point for him. The exciting news was to come from the mother of one of the patients, the patient whose bed was next to Chuck's. He was a young man who had stoned himself out of his head with LSD and was not recovering. He did little but stare out into space. His mother was a pleasant woman, poorly dressed and diffident. She was there to try to help. Chuck knew that the prognosis was pathetic and that the mother was wasting her time, so he tried to be kind to her and hoped to involve her in friendly conversation.

His conversations with her were an exercise in futility until one particular matter was brought to the group. It was a problem connected with a sullen, miserable young woman who was in her mid-twenties, and who had been driven out of her gourd by her dominating religious mother. That mother was there too, and said something about her daughter—something of a religious nature. This got a "tut-tut" from the psychiatrist who was running the session. The "tut-tut" wasn't very strong, and so at this point the boy's mother spoke up.

"We have to learn to separate Christ from Christianity. He is what rescues us, not some religious point of view."

This drew far more than a "tut-tut." The doctor came down hard. "We do not discuss that kind of thing in this hospital. We are interested in reality and a return to the real world. That religious concept is only for those who are outside. We don't bring such things into this hospital. In here we have only a scientific orientation."

The woman looked abashed, and Chuck decided to talk to her again when the session was over and try to ease the blow. It seemed wise to bide his time. It might be better if the psychiatrist did not see him talking to the woman. He waited until the man was busy with someone else. At an opportune moment he spoke to her.

"I agree with what you said, what you said about Christ. Are you a Christian?"

"Yes." She spoke a little hestitantly. It is not always good to have someone agree with you who has been certified as insane.

"Do you attend a Church?"

She answered reluctantly. "Yes, I go to a Pentecostal church."

Chuck smiled. "I do too, and I think that that is the main reason why I'm in here."

Her eyebrows went up and her attitude changed. She knew Chuck had been a doctor but she had no idea he'd have had anything to do with Pentecostals. She was delighted. "Oh, Dr. Sweigard, there's another doctor in this hospital who has received the Baptism. I think he came to the United States from somewhere in the Far East, and he's connected with the medical school. He does his work here. I've been told that he has the gift of healing."

"Is he a psychiatrist?"

"No."

"Do you know his specialty?"

"I think it has something to do with stomach problems."

"What's his name."

"Dr. Kan Uyeyama."

Chuck caught the doctor eyeing them, and gently changed the subject. But he resolved he'd find that doctor if he could, as soon as he could, and went looking for him that afternoon. He found the right part of the hospital and to his relief it was a part that was accessible to him, but he was told that Dr. Uyeyama was not in on Mondays. Tuesday afternoon, as soon as Chuck was free enough to slip away, he went looking again. He found the young doctor in a small individual lab. It was full of equipment and Dr. Uyeyama was using some of it as he worked on a piece of tissue. Chuck knew right away that the man was not in good standing with the administration. Those who stand in well with the powers that be are not given labs that have bars on the windows.

"Doctor," Chuck asked, "may I speak to you?"

Kan Uyeyama looked up from his work and took in Chuck with just one glance. It was obvious that the man was from the Psych ward. "Certainly. What do you want?"

Chuck liked the voice and he wanted badly to really see the man. With great effort, he worked at pulling his eyes into focus and for a moment he succeeded. He got a clear look at the small oriental doctor in front of him. Then his vision fuzzed again. "Doctor, I've been told by a visitor in one of our group therapy sessions that you are a Christian and a Pentecostal."

"Yes." Kan was suddenly cautious. From some of his colleagues he'd taken some teasing that had been unkind, and it paid to be discreet. This man in front of him was sick, and the doctor had no way of knowing what was coming next. The patient could be a set up for the purpose of further embarrassment to Kan.

Chuck felt the tension and understood it. He spoke quietly. "I'm a Pentecostal too."

"That's nice."

"I'm also a doctor. I'm Charles Sweigard, M.D."

Kan's attitude changed immediately. "I heard that they had an M.D. in that snake pit. How did you get in there?"

"Could I sit down while I tell you?"

Kan was immediately solicitous. "Please do." He took hold of the one lab stool available and placed it in a convenient spot. "You seem to be suffering from Akithesia."

"I am. My whole twisted spine is a side effect of the combination of prolixin and some other drugs. The only way to relieve the pain is to lie down, or if you're walking, to throw your rear end backward and take the pressure off the spine. This position has been used by my doctor as an evidence of latent homosexuality."

Dr. Uyeyama snorted. "Tell me the real story."

Chuck did. It was a relief to tell it, and to tell it to a believing and understanding listener. That hadn't happened on a one-to-one basis since he'd talked to the milkman, Jim. When he was finished, Kan asked a question.

"What is God doing? Why do you think He has left you in this place?"

"I'm probably in here for several reasons, one of which I think is obvious. Humiliation and suffering tend to change one's perspective."

"That's a beautiful spirit. I'm not sure I'd have it if I were going through what you're going through. May God bless you. How can I help?"

"Two ways. First I hear that you're gifted with healing."

"I would not go that far. I have prayed for some patients and they have gotten well. I was a joke around here, my praying was a joke, until a couple of good solid stomach cancer patients walked out of the hospital twenty-four hours after I'd prayed for them. The laughter ceased and has been replaced by a mystified silence. No one mentions those cases, and my colleagues tend to keep me at arm's length."

"I know the feeling," Chuck remarked with a grimace. "Would you pray for me? These side effects are getting to me, and the constipation has wrecked me. What hurts even more is my loss of clear vision. My eyes are what they were before I met the Lord, only worse. It's as though God has taken away the sign of His presence."

Kan looked out into the hall. No one was in sight. He stepped back into his cubicle and closed the curtain. He prayed. Chuck felt relief welling up in his soul as someone spoke to God on his behalf. It was good to know that he wasn't the only human being in the hospital on that frequency, and some of his acute loneliness fell away. Whether or not there would be any physical changes, the prayer was a comfort.

When he was through praying, Kan made an offer. "Do you want me to get you some drugs?"

"No. Don't take that chance. I expect to go home to Modesto with my wife for the week end, leaving Friday afternoon. I have a pharmacist friend there who will help me out with whatever I want. It is better if you don't violate the rules so flagrantly. But there is one rule you can violate if you will. It is my second request."

"What is it?"

"I need desperately to lie down. They don't let us do it in the day time. The theory is it might interfere with our sleep the following night. When I can only sit or walk, ultimately I'm in severe pain. It's getting to me."

Kan pointed to a long padded seat built into the corner of the lab. "I stretch out on that once in a while. Let me get the books and papers off it."

In a few seconds there was a place to lie down. Kan picked up a loose leaf note book and placed it on the lab table near his microscope. "This is a paper on which I am working. If someone comes along and I have to wake you, get to your feet and look at the notebook. I will start talking to you about it. It contains a complex problem. That way, if someone puts their head past the curtain, we will be busy looking at a medical problem. Now go to sleep. If no one comes, I'll let you sleep for an hour. Then you'd better go back to your chamber of horrors before you're missed for too long a time. And come back up here tomorrow if you can get away."

Chuck put his head down, grateful to Kan and grateful to God. He had been getting close to the end of his rope. The sleep would make a world of difference. It would give him strength for the next battle.

Best of all, better than anything that had happened to him for months, he had found a friend and a brother in Christ.

PART V

22 Oct 65
San Francisco

Chuck's knowledge of psychiatry was still making him his own worst enemy. He knew too much in one way, and not enough in another, but he was learning. He was learning that that which is untranslatable is untranslatable, leave it alone. Every time he lost an argument, and he lost a lot of them, the words of Jesus would come crashing down the corridors of his mind, "Except a man be born again, he cannot see the kingdom of God."

That was a true statement, and because the psychiatrist was not born again he could not see. There was no way to describe regeneration in psychological terms, only the psychological factors of regeneration could be described. Describing these was a futile process. It was like telling a man that a cube is composed of six squares when he lives in a world that has only two dimensions. Chuck's attempts to reduce spiritual things to only psychological phenomenon had ended in nothing but disaster time after time.

The temptation to try to explain the inexplicable was strongest during group sessions. Chuck suspected that this was true because there was an ego involvement. He had no desire to be thought of as crazy. It was now going to get worse, for the temptation to the ego trip was going to be made stronger by the presence of Cathy. It was bad enough to be where he was always trying to justify his position, it was going to be worse to be in that position in her presence. He should maintain a noncommittal, bland kind of conversation, but he wasn't sure he'd be able to do so no matter how hard he tried.

As it turned out, her presence made matters even worse than he had anticipated. She came to the session as the suffering spouse of a deranged husband. In her own eyes, this was what she was. What added fuel to that fire was the fact that the psychiatrist saw her as she saw herself. He and Cathy made quite a team, and for Chuck, the session went badly.

She asked Chuck a question which, from her point of view, could be considered a very reasonable question. "When are you going to admit you've had hallucinations?"

The psychiatrist interrupted, "I'm sorry, Mrs. Sweigard . . ."

She interrupted, "Call me Cathy."

"Thank you. I'm sorry Cathy but we don't usually use that word in this connection. The medical term for what your husband has is 'fixed delusion.' He simply is not yet willing to come to terms with the real world and let go of his fixed delusion. But I think progress is being made."

The only progress that Chuck was aware of, was his growing ability to hold his tongue and not argue so much. His was a balance difficult to maintain. He couldn't "clam up" without facing the possibility of shock treatments. He couldn't express his religious experiences in psychological terms, and he was handicapped by the intake of mind dulling drugs. All the cards were in the other hand. All but one.

A verse had come back to him out of his earlier reading in the New Testament. It was in the book of Philippians. ". . . wherefore God has given Him a name that is above every name, that at the name of Jesus every knee should bow . . ." Chuck had begun to use that name. When he couldn't handle the surroundings, when he couldn't handle the nagging questions, when he couldn't handle the pain and the boredom, he could say silently to himself, over and over again, "Jesus, Jesus, Jesus . . ."

He was doing it now with part of his mind while he tried to think of something to say. He was relieved of the necessity by Cathy's next question to the psychiatrist.

"Doctor, if my husband were to give up this fixed delusion do you think he would get well?"

"I certainly do."

"And he could go back to practicing medicine and to making a living?"

The psychiatrist was delighted. Chuck had been a problem to him. He could see that now he was going to get some needed help. "I'm quite sure of it, Cathy. Nothing is absolutely concrete in any field of medicine, including psychiatry, and we can be disappointed, but in my professional opinion, were your husband to give up his fixed delusion he would be practicing medicine successfully in a matter of months."

Cathy had heard just what she wanted Chuck to hear. She said, "Thank you, doctor."

PART VI

Their drive from San Francisco to Modesto began in silence and continued in silence. This was no hardship for Chuck, he delighted in it. He was getting a little stronger in both mind and body. He owed this improvement to reduced medication. The reduction was not the doctor's idea, but Chuck's. They no longer gave him shots, but oral medication, and he was becoming an expert at getting some of the pills back out of his mouth unobtrusively. He couldn't spit them all out, the side effects of the medicine would disappear and they would know what he was doing. They'd soon have him back on shots. He settled for two-thirds of the prescriptions by spitting out one pill in every three. He had "palmed" all of Friday's medication and so his thinking ability—and God be praised—his vision were clearing up.

Under ordinary circumstances the scenery would be nothing to brag about, in the fall the hills are brown or barren, but to Chuck they looked lovely and when they topped the rise and looked down into the valley he could see for miles. The most beautiful part of the view was the fact that he didn't have to look through bars to see it.

The continued silence was not easy for Cathy to take. By the time they reached the town of Tracy she could take it no longer, and asked the question that was burning a hole in her gut. "For the sake of us all, are you going to do what the doctor said and give up your delusion?"

Chuck was silent for a moment, and then when

he answered he seemed to change the subject. "Remember when we were married?"

Cathy spoke with great bitterness. "I certainly do. I've thought about it many times."

"You didn't get whom you wanted, did you? I was your second choice."

She put her bottom lip between her teeth for a moment before she answered. "You finally figured that out."

"I didn't figure that out. Several months ago, you left the morning paper on the kitchen table folded in such a way that Mike's picture was prominently displayed. He was coming to Modesto to lecture at Doctor's Hospital, and there was an article about it. When I looked at that picture, I knew you had been looking at it too, and the light came on." He turned toward her. "Cathy, you are and you were beautiful. You were literally the sweetheart of Sigma Chi. Why didn't you marry Mike? He too was on his way to being a doctor. He's been very successful."

Cathy was driving. She had to drive; she was the only one with a valid driver's license. She stopped the station wagon for the one red light in Tracy. Then she turned and looked at Chuck when she answered. Their eyes met.

"He wouldn't ask me."

"I would think that you would have been able to talk him into it."

"I tried, believe me I tried. When that didn't work, I asked him to marry me. I almost did it on my knees. He said no."

The traffic light turned green, she put her eyes back on the road and her foot touched the accelerator. East of Tracy, highway 32 would turn south and she'd follow it into Modesto. Chuck was silent for a few moments before he spoke again.

"So, Mike had turned you down, then when I asked you, you said yes. You couldn't get doctor number one, so you took doctor number two."

"That's the picture."

"That's not the whole picture. I've been doing some thinking. There's time to think when you're incarcerated, provided you're not too doped to do it."

This conversation hadn't gone the way Cathy wanted it to, not at all. If when it had started she'd known where it was going to go, she would have endured the silence. Chuck continued.

"After my conversion, or if you prefer, after my first delusion, when I could really make love to you the way a man should, you didn't like it because you wished, and you still wish, that I were someone else."

"That's the way it is; what are you going to do about it?"

"Nothing. I gave my word, ' . . . for better or for worse, in sickness and in health. . .' and I'll keep my word."

"I've kept my word too; I've never let anyone else touch me."

"No, you haven't kept your word. You promised to love me, and that you have never done."

Cathy was crying. Chuck wished from the

depths of his soul that her tears might turn into tears of sorrow. If they did, they could have some fellowship some day, but he knew they were not shed in sorrow. They were shed in anger, anger that showed through in the hate and bitterness in her voice.

"God knows I tried."

"All right, try something else. When we were married in that three hundred year old chapel in Pennsylvania, we were the ideal, happy, handsome couple. At that time we both said we believed in God. Do you still believe in Him?"

"I don't know for sure, but I think so."

"Then why don't you pray and ask God whether or not I'm crazy?"

The fury of her response let him know he'd gone too far. She pointed back toward the late afternoon sun getting lower in the sky behind them. "Do you see that sun?"

"Yes."

"Turn around and take a good look at it." He did as he was told and she continued. "Should I pray and ask God whether or not the sun is shining? How stupid can you be? A half a dozen psychiatrists, a judge, the whole State of California says Charles B. Sweigard is nuts. Why in the world would I ask God about that?"

"Because they are wrong, I'm not nuts."

Ahead of them, there was a farm house the front yard of which made a wide spot in the road. The wide spot was there for a reason. A large sign in front of the house said, FRESH EGGS, and behind the house there were hen houses. Cathy took advantage of the wide spot and pulled off the road. She killed her engine and turned and looked at Chuck again.

"I can prove you're crazy."

The ventilation system turned off as the engine died. Chuck rolled down his window before he answered her. "How?"

"Do you like it at Langley Porter?"

"Of course not."

"Do you want to get out?"

"More than anything in the world."

"You can get out. All you have to do is to say to that young psychiatrist, 'I have had a delusion, I see that now,' and he'd dismiss you so fast it would make your head swim. He'd call you a cure and happily take credit for it. Then, after you were home, you would be free to believe anything you wanted to believe. Now wouldn't a sane man do it?"

Chuck smiled. "The temptation is great, believe me. It crosses my mind ten times a day."

"Why don't you do it, if you're sane?"

Chuck pointed to the farm house. It was weatherbeaten and in need of paint and repair. The yard around it needed attention. Apparently time and effort went into chickens. "Did you hear that rooster?"

"What rooster?"

"The one that just crowed."

"No."

"I did."

"What has that got to do with what we're talking about?"

"Two thousand years ago, a man named Peter who knew Jesus and knew that He was the Christ denied three times that he had ever met Him. Then a cock crowed. Peter wept and then he was forgiven. After a while he even forgave himself, but Peter was lucky. His denial preceded the giving of the Holy Spirit. I'm on the other side of Pentecost, I have the Holy Spirit. If I deny that I met Jesus in that kitchen that night, the night I wanted to commit suicide, someday, before my heavenly Father, Jesus may have to deny that He ever knew me. If that happened, I might hear that cock that just crowed, hear it in hell forever."

Cathy started the engine and eased the car back on to the road. "Let's say that the story is true, the story about Christ, that He did die and rise from the dead. Let's say it is historic fact, I don't know for sure whether it is or not, but supposing it is. Do you want me to believe that this same God-man met Chuck Sweigard one night and told him not to commit suicide, that this same Jesus spanned the distance from Palestine to California, and spanned two thousand years of time and showed up in our kitchen in Modesto and had a conversation with you? You are balmy."

The verse came back to Chuck. "Except a man be born again, he can not see the kingdom of God." Apparently, that applied to women too. Chuck made the mistake of saying so and a near violent and completely pointless argument continued all the way to Modesto. All of Chuck's high standards of spiritual insight and understanding, all his desire to be sweetly reasonable disappeared into the maelstrom of domestic warfare.

CHAPTER SIX

Robert L. Hill, M.D.   *Practice Limited*
                                          to Psychiatry

Re: Charles B. Sweigard, Jr., M.D.

". . . his wife, who suffers from a tendency to be generally anxious, was made uneasy by his (Chuck's) newly found faith and tended to see it in pathological terms. This accounts for important miscommunications. For example, he never had the impression he was the Messiah, nor did he have the fear of dying that are noted in hospital records, such history being distorted moderately by third parties. . ."

PART I

SAN FRANCISCO

More than a month had gone by since Chuck had met Kan. The Japanese doctor had been a godsend, but he was not enough. The time that Chuck spent in Kan's lab, he spent sleeping. He needed the sleep if he were to hold his act together, but if in addition to the sleep he were to take time from Kan for fellowship, he would be imposing unreasonably. Kan's time in his lab was limited and he was there to produce results as a result of lab work. He couldn't get those results if he spent an hour a day in fellowship with Chuck.

Sweigard was feeling blue. It was a Monday and that was the worst day of the week because of the three days that preceded it. Friday had contained another miserable group session in which the psychiatrist and Cathy ganged up on him. This was followed by a Saturday and Sunday at home in Modesto, if you could call a bitter, two-day diatribe a visit at "home." He needed to talk to someone, someone who would understand.

Chuck was sitting on his bed, feeling sorry for himself, and with difficulty keeping his eyes dry. He didn't dare shed tears. They would not go unobserved. At Langley Porter, there were nurses and attendants at a ratio of two to one over patients. Almost everything was observed. Openly shed tears would be evidence of regression and in his case that would mean increased medication which he did not want. He set his teeth and prayed silently. "Jesus, send someone to talk to me."

His prayer was answered the next day. A man walked into the ward who looked vaguely familiar. Although Chuck couldn't remember where he had seen him, he knew his profession as soon as he looked at him. The man wore a black suit, black shoes, white shirt and black tie. His hair was gray, and under his arm, without so much as a by-your-leave, he carried a large black-bound King James

Bible. He was a Pentecostal minister, and that was something that Chuck never expected to see in the ward at Langley Porter, except perhaps as a patient.

The preacher walked over to Chuck and put out his hand. "Dr. Sweigard, it is good to see you again. I'm Pastor Jones."

"I'm glad to see you, but where have we met?" Chuck had gotten up off his bed awkwardly to greet the man and shake hands with him.

"Please, keep your seat, doctor. Make yourself as comfortable as possible." Chuck sat back down on his bed, and the pastor sat down beside him before he continued talking. "I was introduced to you by Brother Jim. I was visiting the Modesto church the night you came forward to receive the baptism."

"Where's your church and how in the world did you get in here?"

The man held up his hand. "Easy, brother, one question at a time. I'm from Visalia."

"That's a hundred miles from here."

"I know. This morning I was praying for you, I'd heard from brother Jim that you were in here because of your faith, and the Lord laid it on my heart to come see you. I knew I was to come right away, it was a very strong leading. When I got here, I walked into the building with some other people, and no one asked me a thing. I just came on upstairs."

"With that Bible under your arm?"

"Yes."

"How did you know where to come?"

"The Lord wanted me here, so I just knew."

"I'm glad you're here and I'm amazed, I asked God yesterday for someone to talk to, someone who would understand."

Chuck was amazed about something else too. Nurses, attendants, and doctors should have been around them like swarming bees. This did not happen. It was as though no one could see them. Chuck had a mild case of goose flesh.

"God has given me a message for you, brother." The man opened his King James to where he had put his marker. The marker was a small, hand-crocheted cross. "The Gospel of Matthew the tenth chapter and the sixteenth verse." Although Jones kept his voice down, his mannerisms were those of a man addressing a crowd of thousands. 'Behold, I send you forth as sheep in the midst of wolves: be ye therefore wise as serpents, and harmless as doves.' Brother, I expect you're harmless enough in here. They would see to that, but I wonder if you are being wise. Are you trying to testify?"

"Not really. I'm just trying to keep them from labeling me crazy, and I'm trying to keep from denying my Lord."

"The second thing is commendable, but I'm not sure about the first. Why shouldn't they think you are crazy? Does not Paul say that the Gospel is foolishness to those who are perishing? Are you going to change that with your wisdom?"

Chuck was abashed. "In my better moments, I know this, but I can't keep my mouth shut."

"You must do so, Brother, or you'll be here forever. Let them think whatever they want to think. Do not encourage that which is false, but do not try to change it. That is not your responsibility. Your responsibility is to get out of here and do the work that God will call you to do. When you are tempted to speak, remember the words of our Lord. He has forbidden us to cast pearls before swine. In here, they will indeed trample them in the mud and turn and rend you. You cannot preach the Gospel in this place."

Chuck felt humbled. He doubted that this man had anything more than a high school education, if he had that much, so he might be very short on knowledge, but he was obviously not short on wisdom.

"Pastor Jones, will you pray for me?"

The Pentecostal pastor did, quietly and in King James English. Chuck found it a blessing and he wanted more. "Thank you for that prayer. Can you stay for a while?"

"No. The Spirit is telling me to leave."

"Can you come back?"

"Only if the Spirit sends me. I would never get in this place unless He prepared the way. This is Satan's domain."

Chuck watched him leave as he had come, walking out as though he owned the place, with his Bible prominently displayed under his arm, completely and inexplicably ignored by all who saw him. He came again in about ten days. They had some more fellowship, and another word of prayer. Then Pastor Jones left for the second time and Chuck never saw him again.

Pastor Jones' visits were followed by a change in Chuck. He soon made a move that divided the forces against him. At a group therapy session when Cathy was present, he brought up the important subject—money. Chuck's insurance was reaching its limits, the policy was not going to pay the 75% of his salary it had been paying, time was running out. If he stayed in the hospital much longer, he was going to face bankruptcy.

This had a remarkable effect on Cathy. It was suddenly more important for her husband to get well and start earning a living, than it was for the world to confirm her opinion of the fact that he was crazy. So, when the psychiatrist asked her how the previous week end had gone, her tune changed. It seemed that Chuck was improving. They had had severe arguments, but Chuck hadn't been the casper milque toast of the past, he had stood up and made his point heard. Chuck started to ask how violent arguments could be a sign of increasing mental health, but then he remembered Pastor Jones and kept his mouth shut. He'd let them believe what they wanted to believe.

The psychiatrist was impressed. Cathy seemed so level-headed and capable of handling the situation, that he asked her if she thought Chuck could be taken care of at home. Cathy was not delighted with the idea, but if he were home instead of being institutionalized, he'd be that much closer to earning an income. It was not as though she had to call her husband cured, treatment would continue. She would have to come back to the Langley Porter Hospital with him twice a week for group therapy sessions. If, under that arrangement, Chuck continued to "improve" he might expect complete rehabilitation.

All this sounded fine, but Chuck knew better. He could hope to get a certificate of competence and be re-admitted to the practice of medicine, but complete rehabilitation was not something that came easily or quickly, if it ever came at all. Once a man had served time in a prison for a felony, he would remain under suspicion after he got out. If a man was declared legally insane, the onus was on him for years if not for life.

January 17, 1966 came and with it came liberty. Chuck and Cathy had agreed to place themselves under the care of Dr. Robert Hill in Stockton. Chuck liked Dr. Hill and happily exchanged him for treatment at Langley Porter. Also he liked the idea of going to Stockton for treatment. It could have proved embarrassing to have had to use someone in Modesto. And so Chuck left Langley Porter with a certificate of competency in his hand, looking forward to his appointment to meet with the committee of the Stanislaus County Medical Association. He'd soon be practicing medicine again.

Outside the institution, getting ready to get into his car, and this time, drive it, with his hand on the door handle he looked back at the building, which for him had been the front porch of hell for months. He believed that he would never be in one of those again, that he would never be under an institutional psychiatrist, and that he would never again be committed. He was wrong on all three counts.

PART II

THE LANGLEY PORTER
NEUROPSYCHIATRIC INSTITUTE

DISCHARGE SUMMARY

Sweigard, Charles, B., Jr.
LPNI No. 6928

RECOMMENDATIONS: The patient and his wife
both eagerly accepted recommendation for follow-up
private therapy with Dr. Robert Hill, Stockton, California.

4 Feb 66
MODESTO

It was Friday and the end of Chuck's week of
work at the Medical Group. His name was back on
the curb marking his parking place and he was back
into the full swing of things. His practice was building up again fast. He liked children and they liked
him, and his looks and his manner set well with
their mothers. He was bringing home two thousand
dollars a month and the Sweigards would soon be
out of debt. They had sold their second house and
moved into a still smaller one. That had moved the
children to different schools yet again, and again in
the middle of a year. But things were getting better.
They would soon be able to afford a larger house,

and maybe this time Cathy would help choose and not just stand back in anger.

They were getting along a little better. It was something like an armed truce. No open warfare, but things were kept at arm's length and no communication with his children was permitted, not about "the religious ideas that had caused his sickness."

The next few weeks were an almost happy time. Being out of the hospital was a source of joy, and he was finding that time spent with Dr. Hill was not wasted time. The psychiatrist was good and the sessions helpful. No one is totally "normal," there are personality problems in everybody, and Chuck had his. Dr. Hill was a help. Chuck's childhood had not been completely happy and he had carried some scars. The psychiatrist did some digging and got to the bottom of one or two problems.

It was during one of these sessions that Dr. Hill asked him about the hospitalization for psychiatric reasons while in medical school. Chuck insisted that he had not been hospitalized. Dr. Hill showed him the report in his hospital records that said he had been hospitalized. He also showed him the remark that psychiatric attention had been suggested while Chuck was on duty in Japan. Dr. Hill had brought these matters up during a session in which Cathy was not present and the two doctors were alone. Chuck assured him that the source of both pieces of misinformation had to be Cathy. They had probably gotten into the record through the minister friend. Hill promised to add a letter to his file that would clear both matters.

That was not the only correction that the psychiatrist made in Chuck's records. He was firmly convinced that Chuck had been badly diagnosed at Stockton and said so, in writing, to the California Board of Medical Examiners.

Things did not go equally well during Cathy's visits. As he had done before, Dr. Hill tried to bring her around to where she could see that she was making her contributions to the problems. She would not or could not see this and she would liked to have stopped seeing him, but she was in a box. Without the continuing therapy, the Board of Medical Examiners might not be happy about leaving Chuck his license. Without the license there would be no income. Cathy would put up with a lot to get back into the swing of things. New clothes, new cars, and new houses all cost money. She'd put up with Hill and his questions, but she contributed little to the sessions she attended.

Only once did she break out of her mold. She pointed out that the psychiatrist at Langley Porter had treated her differently than Dr. Hill did. His reply had been short and sweet.

"I do not share that man's diagnosis of your husband. I think he was wrong." The matter was not broached again.

Then the axe fell. In the midst of this, Chuck got a second call from Bert, who was still the president of the Group. The hatchet jobs were still his department. Like the first call, this one came at night, but there were two differences between the calls. The first one had been expected, the second one was a surprise; the first one had left Chuck with options.

This one didn't; it was cold turkey.

"Chuck, Bert here." The voice was officious and unfriendly.

"Yes, sir." He felt his stomach sink a little.

"We've been going over your record since you rejoined us. There seems to be quite a little lab work ordered for your patients, more than other doctors demand. As you know you're one of three pediatricians with The Group and that gives us a basis for comparison."

Chuck didn't say anything. He knew that that wasn't the real problem. He knew that Bert knew that on three occasions some lab work ordered had resulted in his finding something that did a great deal for the little patient, something that had been passed up by someone else. There was no point in calling attention to this when Bert knew it already. Bert ran the place with an iron hand and never missed a trick. Chuck held his silence.

Bert cleared his throat, he had been waiting for a protest that didn't come. "Another thing is that you seem to spend more time with a patient than do the other pediatricians."

This was getting closer to the truth. Some of the time spent with some of his patients had been time used to talk about the Lord or to pray about something. Chuck was sure that this was thought of as "unscientific" and resented by several of the doctors. Chuck decided to present matters to Bert on the basis of Bert's value judgements.

"I happen to have looked at the books on my last completed month's work. If you multiply that month's gross by twelve months, it comes out to over eighty thousand dollars a year. You're paying me twenty-four thousand plus benefits. That's a mark up to you on my work of about fifty-six thousand dollars. I have to have been seeing patients, or the dollars wouldn't be there."

This was not the argument that Bert had expected and there was another silence. However, he was equal to the occasion. "That's true, but if we give your spot to someone equally talented, we'll make even more won't we?"

The chances of finding someone else who would match his gross were not probable and Chuck knew it. He knew Bert knew it. The matter boiled down to two things. In Chuck they had a doctor who had been institutionalized and was under psychiatric care. This was embarrassing. Worse, they had a doctor who was a religious nut and prayed with his patients.

Bert finished the conversation with a reminder. "I suggest you look at your contract, Dr. Sweigard. When you signed it, you agreed not to practice medicine within one hundred miles of here if you left our Group."

Chuck didn't answer, he just hung up. When he got a dial tone again he called one of the two pediatricians who practiced with him at the Group. This one, Dr. Robert Elliot, was kindly disposed toward Chuck and openly admired Chuck's medicine. Chuck dialed Elliot's unlisted home number and got his colleague after only one ring. "Bob, this is Chuck Sweigard."

"Hi! Problem?"

"Yes. I just got fired."

"What! Come off it. Who told you?"

"Bert himself. They'll have the notice on my desk the next time I go in. It will all be spelled out in nice legal terminology, but it will be the same thing. I'm still fired."

"Why?"

"The real reasons were not mentioned, but I think that my psychiatric record is an embarrassment, and my testimony is worse."

"I warned you about that. There are some stinkers we work with who think that no intelligent person has believed in a personal God since the Neanderthal man. Do you have any plans? What are you going to do?"

"Bert gave me the word that I'd have to move a hundred miles away. I hate that, my kids have already gone from pillar to post."

"Hey! I can help you there." Bob had a little jubilation in his voice. "I checked that out with an attorney before I signed it, and I've been told that it won't stand up in court. Don't take my word for it, find your own attorney, but the picture seems to be that if you do very well, and leave the Group and take your patients with you, they can give you trouble. But, if they tell you that you are unsatisfactory and that you are to leave, they can't make it stick. Do you want to practice around here?"

"Yes."

"Then it might interest you to know that there is a big vacancy in the Stark Dental Building."

"Where is that?"

"It's on the south side of McHenry just east of the bridge, three or four blocks before you get to Morris. It's half a dozen small buildings made of stucco and trimmed in brick with a red tile roof. The center suite is the largest and the dentist that had it has moved out. It shouldn't cost too much to alter it for a pediatrician. If you settle there, I'll be glad to drop a hint or two to some of your patients when they get shifted to me. It won't take you long to build a practice."

"Thank you, Bob. You've eased a blow."

Chuck was in practice for himself within two weeks, and many of his former patients followed him. He acted as both doctor and nurse. The only employee was a girl who answered the phone, made appointments, greeted patients, and kept the books. She worked out fine. Her big drawback didn't show up until later. She developed an affinity for Cathy Sweigard and as they became friends, Chuck began to play "odd man out" but at first there was no problem.

Within two weeks of his office opening, one month after he had left the group, he was busy and he had a decent income. Then he began to feel ill at ease. Many of those who brought their children to him, had definite ideas of how their child should be treated, and what the diagnosis should be. It is a common form of parental manipulation. They thought that a doctor setting up a single practice would need their business and do what they wanted. He didn't want to practice that kind of medicine. He began to pray about it.

The answers to his prayers were quick. First, new patients came, those for whom the county paid. The county didn't pay much but it paid something. They contrasted with a few of his wealthy patients who thought doctors should be happy with them as patients even if they never got around to paying anything. The charity patients were low pay but they brought something with them that Chuck liked, they brought a challenge, they brought problems that were not easily solved. He discovered that in some cases the child had been badly misdiagnosed. He didn't think the cause of this was incompetence as much as it was haste. Some doctors with an eye on their income don't usually want to spend time and money digging too deeply into the problems of county patients.

This began to change Chuck's method of practicing medicine. His personal experience with the tie-in between body, mind and spirit gave him insight. He understood suffering and illness as few doctors do and he began to use a whole person approach. He put together a questionnaire that would bring to light what he wanted to know about a new patient, and he knew where he was apt to be going before medical treatment started. This led to some remarkable changes in patients and in recoveries of all kinds, including recovery from spiritual illness. More than one patient and more than one patient's parent came to a belief in and committal to Jesus Christ. Chuck was as happy as he'd ever been, and delighted with his practice. It was at this point that the bubble broke.

The friendly conversations between his wife and his secretary ended the trucc with a bang. The secretary mentioned in passing that it was wonderful that a doctor of Charles Sweigard's enormous ability would be willing not only to spend time with county patients, but to work with those who couldn't pay at all. The telephone conversation ended and Cathy was in the office within a few minutes to look at the books. What she saw made her angry enough to have it out right there and then.

From her point of view there was no excuse for what was going on and she said so. The walls between the offices and the waiting room were not all that thick, and Chuck tried to pacify her until they could talk at home.

"Let's talk about it tonight."

"We'll talk about it now. What are you doing? I have no maid, I am behind on my dues at the racquet club, I haven't bought enough in the way of new clothes to mention, not for months, my car is three years old, I live in a house smaller than that of any other doctor's wife I know of, your children go to one of the poorer schools in town, we have little or nothing in the savings, and you are sitting in your office treating patients who can't pay. Haven't you ever heard of public clincis?"

"Yes, and I've had a personal taste of public supported medicine and it wasn't all that satisfying. I don't always recommend it."

"Well, isn't that too bad! What about your own family? How do you want us to live? If I had wanted to live like we're living I could have married a bus driver. I married a doctor, but no one can tell that by looking at the way we live! You just don't care about us at all, you're religious and you're insane and that's the worst possible combination."

"I'll talk to you about it tonight."

"I'll be there tonight and we'll talk about it, we're not going to talk about anything else until you change." She leaned across the desk and put her face near his and yelled. "Make some money!"

She left, but she left disaster behind her. In a small town, professional people live in glass houses. When there is a domestic quarrel, word gets around. People know that there is apt to be trouble ahead. This belief influences credit, it has an effect on relationships with colleagues, and it has its effect on a practice. Doctors on their way to a nasty divorce don't always have their minds on the medicine they're practicing. In addition to all this, there is an antagonism built into that kind of a society, an antagonism to marital wars in general and to those fought in public in particular.

This war was fought in public. Cathy came to the office daily. She studied the books and sent out bills and stiff demands on them. Some bills she turned over to a collection agency. She was very polite to paid up patients and short with the others. The practice was down to half of what it had been in a matter of weeks. Chuck was getting to the end of his rope.

PART III

State of California
DEPARTMENT OF MENTAL HYGIENE
Release Summary   *Sweigard, Charles B.*
          MODESTO STATE HOSPITAL
                    MOD 025280

Date of Admission 8-4-66

COURSE IN HOSPITAL:
Patient had to be removed bodily from his office as he would not assist in anyway. On arrival at hospital he remained extremely limp, semicatatonic and passive and had to be brought in by wheelchair. He was preoccupied with relating his religious experiences.

4 Aug 66
MODESTO

It was Thursday noon. Chuck sat at his desk praying. The fight at home had intensified, and he could not make himself maintain a prudent silence. He had deteriorated to the place where he joined the fray willingly, and he knew that this was wrong. There was no possibility of winning Cathy over by fighting with her. He wouldn't be able to affect her thinking through persuasion, much less by argument. He knew now that he should never have tried. He should have backed off, way off, and prayed. If he had said nothing to his wife about God and a great deal about his wife to God, things might not have reached their impasse.

This was his third day of fasting and prayer. He prayed whenever he could arrange it and he was praying during his lunch hour. His Bible was on his desk beside his elbow and he had started to pick it up and read it, but his hand stopped in mid-air. He knew that he was in for another experience. The feeling of complete peace came over him and an insight was given, an insight into the sovereignty of God. Chuck saw the world, the very little world, held in loving, tender hands. A feeling of total acceptance and a sense of separation from everything around him let him know that a day would come when he would step out of this world and into the next and into an all-encompassing love.

He continued to sit at his desk quietly weeping because of an inexplicable inner joy and a sense of the Lord's presence with him. That was the moment that Cathy entered the room on one of her unannounced visits. She saw the strange mixture of peace and tears on his face.

"What's the matter?"

He answered her in a very kind way. "Nothing is the matter, abolutely nothing. You may say anything you wish to say, the peace that I'm experiencing right now will stay intact." He opened his desk drawer and pulled out a rather large pin. He pushed it into his arm. "See that? No pain, no unpleasantness. Right now no matter what anyone said it would not hurt. My soul is just like my body."

Cathy was scared. She saw the Bible on his desk and she picked it up. "Maybe, if I read something from this, it would cheer you up."

"Nothing could cheer me more than I'm cheered right now, but if you would like to read something, go right ahead."

She opened the Bible to the New Testament. Matthew 12:23 happened to be at the top of the page and she began to read it. From her point of view, it started out appropriately enough. "Then a blind and dumb demoniac was brought to him and he healed him, so that the dumb man spoke and saw. And all the people were amazed and said, 'Can this be the Son of David?' But when the Pharisees heard it they said, 'It is only by Beelzebul, the prince of demons, that this man casts out demons.' Knowing their thoughts, he said to them, 'Every kingdom divided against itself is laid waste and no city or house . . .'" at that point she choked. She tried again, "and no city or house . . ."

"Let me finish it for you," Chuck interjected quietly. "No house divided against itself can stand."

Cathy stood stock still for a moment or two and then turned and walked out. As she left, Chuck's experience ended and he knew that the Lord had prepared him to face the fact that his marriage was over. It had not been a happy marriage, but it had had its moments, and it was a living thing. It also inevitably intertwined the lives of seven people. Divorce is a form of murder. Something that was alive dies, and there is pain. Only those who are separated from reality, only those who take marriage and sex lightly can go through a divorce without bleeding inside.

Chuck called to his secretary. "Marie, I won't

be seeing anyone else today. Get hold of as many patients as you can and tell them not to come. If any come, send them home."

She did as she was told, but as time went by, she began to worry. Chuck had been sitting, staring at the wall for a couple of hours and she was afraid that something was seriously wrong. He had been taken to the state hospital once. She wondered if maybe he should go again. Finally she could stand it no longer and called Cathy.

"This is Marie."

"What's the matter now?" Cathy's voice had an edge to it.

"He's cancelled all appointments and he's sitting staring at the wall. He's been there for hours and I'm scared."

"I'll call Dr. Elliot at the Medical Group, and ask him to drop by and talk to Chuck. They're good friends and Dr. Elliot will know what to do."

"Thank you." There was genuine relief in Marie's voice.

Cathy was wrong. Dr. Elliot didn't know what to do. He listened to Chuck in a courteous and thoughtful manner, but the story sounded weird to him. How could a man see Jesus Christ hold the world in His hands? Worse, the bit about the freedom from pain, the inability to feel a pin when it went into his arm, that sounded bad. Bob Elliot didn't remember much of his psychiatry, he too was a pediatrician, but that didn't sound normal to him. He wanted to consult an expert. This case was not in his field. He excused himself for a moment and went into the lavatory. While in there, he wrote a note to Marie, flushed the toilet for effect, and then went back to where Chuck was sitting. As he passed Marie's desk, he dropped the note on it.

She picked up the paper and read it. "Call the State hospital and have them send an ambulance."

Bob resumed his seat and continued listening to Chuck while he waited for the ambulance. It came quietly and parked in front of the building. The two white clothed attendants were standing one on each side of Chuck before he knew what was happening.

He looked at Bob. "Thanks."

"Chuck, please, I'm not a shrink. I don't know what to do. If you're all right, they'll let you out."

"That's what you think. Besides, the question is academic; I'm not going."

One of the attendants spoke. "I'm sorry, Dr. Sweigard, you're going. I hope you're going quietly, but either way we have to take you."

"All right, I can't win, but I'm not going to help. If you're putting me back into one of those booby hatches, you're going to do all the work. Never again will I walk in voluntarily."

They did all the work. Chuck was a big man and it wasn't easy. He stayed perfectly limp and offered no resistance and no help. It was like trying to move a sack filled with one hundred and eighty pounds of billiard balls. In the end, they succeeded.

At the hospital the unresisting Chuck was placed in a wheelchair. It took four attendants to do it. Then he was wheeled into ADMITTANCE. The young psychiatrist who met him sounded like a brother of the one who had been his doctor at Langley Porter. The questions started again, the same questions. Back to square one. He interrupted the process.

"I am not committing myself, so save yourself the time and the trouble."

The doctor was quite ready to agree. "You don't have to. We'll hold you until we can get our hands on a judge. There are trials for these situations."

"I've been through that charade. You have a judge or two at your mercy. They have no way of knowing that you don't know what you're doing."

"You can look at it that way if you like. Which way are you coming in?"

"I'll commit myself on one condition. I've been reading a book, VARIETIES OF RELIGIOUS EXPERIENCE by James. Someone goes and gets that book and I get to keep it and read it. No one will take it from me until I'm done."

The doctor didn't want the trial if he didn't have to have it. With someone like Sweigard who had been previously committed, the outcome was usually predictable, but it could get sticky. Crazy or sane, Sweigard was smart. "You can have your book."

"I'll sign."

Once more he was in the hands of the State and its doctors.

CHAPTER SEVEN

PART I

State of California
DEPARTMENT OF MENTAL HYGIENE
Release Summary   Sweigard, Charles B.
                MODESTO STATE HOSPITAL
                        MOD 025280

Date of Admission 8-4-66

COURSE IN HOSPITAL . . . After giving up his
limp and passive behavior, he began wandering the
halls, posturing in weird positions. He verbalized con-
tinuously, was preoccupied about his communication
with God, with God's taking care of everything, etc.
He also on repeated occasions was observed to ini-
tiate contact with other male patients, which he de-
nied had any significance . . .

Once admitted and committed, Chuck got up
out of the wheelchair and began to case the place.
The main ward was gross, worse by far than anything he had seen at Langley Porter. The man sitting on the second bed on the right was a toothless,
whizzened evil looking man. As Chuck entered the
ward, the old man pointed at him and gleefully

chuckled. Then he started yelling, over and over, "Jesus lover, mother—; Jesus lover, mother—."

Chuck murmured to himself. "He knows where I'm coming from." The man on the bed next to the man yelling was openly masterbating. "Jesus," Chuck prayed, "please don't make me spend a year in here. Please keep me out of this ward."

His prayers were answered the first night, but not too pleasantly. He was put in a security cell, a bare room with heavy bars on the window. He was given a massive dose of aphenothiazine by injection and in a few minutes was sleepy, so sleepy that he lay down on the floor and slept for twelve hours. When he awoke, he should have been cold, no one had covered him, but he found that he wasn't. He took his warmth and comfort as a gift from the Lord and said his thanks. There was something for which he didn't say thanks; he just groaned, for when he got up off the floor, he discovered that the problem with his back that plagued him at Langley Porter had returned with a vengeance. Just one shot had done it. Once again the pain in his back could be relieved only by throwing his rear out and walking like an arthritic duck.

The door of his cell opened and he was face to face with the head nurse, Gretel. Behind her back she was known as Gratel. Chuck did not hold her hardness against her. No one could assume her responsibilities and not become hard. The alternative was to go crazy and join the inmates. She had a needle in her hand.

"You won't need that. If you're bound and determined to give me the stuff, I'll take the pills."

She shrugged and said, "I'll be back in a minute."

When she returned she had a couple of pills in one hand and a glass of water in the other. She handed it all to Chuck. Something warned him not to play games on this occasion. He swallowed the pills as he drank the water.

Gretel said, "Open your mouth."

He did so, and she ran her finger around his teeth and his tongue and she did it in a way that showed she'd had plenty of practice. The pills, fortunately had been swallowed. If they hadn't, Chuck would have been on the needle for as long as he was there.

PART II

8 Aug 66
MODESTO

God continued to answer Chuck's prayer. He didn't get put into the ward; he had a small room of his own. Tuesday even this was improved and he was placed in something that was almost like a motel suite. He had his own bath and toilet, a closet and a small furnished sitting room. The thing that kept him reminded of where he was were the heavy bars that covered the windows.

He was keeping his medication down to one half of what was prescribed. It was done by a change in "methodology." The pills were palmed, kept in a crack in his hand and never entered his mouth. So, when his mouth was searched it looked like he'd swallowed them. Taking only half gave him the side effects that showed the presence of the medication, but it was a small enough dosage so that he didn't turn into a zombie. There were several of those over-medicated sleep walkers wandering through the halls. He had no desire to join them.

His first confrontation with his psychiatrist had been Monday the eighth, and it had been bad. The young doctor had started asking questions that soon showed prior knowledge of Sweigard's past. Chuck was surprised at the thoroughness of the background knowledge. He hadn't realized he'd revealed so much about himself when he had been at Langley Porter. Then the psychiatrist asked a question that could have been based only on intimate knowledge. It assumed something that he had never told anyone in the world but Cathy. The doctor had been pumping his wife.

During the session they were sitting in the psychiatrist's office, he behind his desk and Chuck in a chair to one side of him. Chuck could see out the window behind the doctor, see the green lawns and people walking around in freedom. As always whenever he looked out he was reminded of where he was. The windows of the doctor's office were no different than any other windows. They too were barred.

"Dr. Sweigard, you're not answering the question."

"For two reasons. You already know the answer, you heard it from my wife, and neither the question nor the answer are any of your business."

"They are my business. I'm your psychiatrist."

"Not a very competent one. If you were you'd know that I'm sane."

"There are ways of showing you that you're not."

"I know them. I went to school too. Just give a patient shock treatments until he'll admit he's anything."

"We don't use shock treatments that way around here."

"That's good, but only because you can do the same thing with chemicals."

"Would you object to truth serum?"

"Violently. I have had a conversion experience. Conversion is a psychological phenomenon. People can be converted to all kinds of things and from all kinds of things; from Fascism to Communism, or Communism to Fascism, but with conversion to Christ, something else can happen which you cannot understand. The New Testament calls it regeneration, which is a term that will make no sense to you unless it happens to you. It means that I have a new nature that is growing, but an old one that isn't dead yet. There are things that can come out of the old nature that I wouldn't want to hear myself saying."

"Like homosexual drives?"

"I have no drives that I know of in that area."

"Strange, two patients in the ward told me that you had made advances."

"They are lying."

The psychiatrist shrugged, picked his pen up off his desk and looked at it as he twirled it in his fingers. "You say that you have two natures. What is the new nature?"

"Jesus Christ. As the New Testament says, 'Christ in you, your hope of glory.'"

"You and Jesus are walking the halls of this institution together then?"

"True to some extent. I wish there were more of Him and less of me."

"And you want me to believe that you're not schizophrenic?"

"If I am, where are the rest of the symptoms?"

"You know enough about psychiatry to hide them."

"I can't win can I?"

"You can't get well either, until you admit you're sick."

"If I did that, I'd be lying. I'm ashamed to say that in a desire to get out of these snake pits, I have tried to lie, but it didn't work. It just confused the issue."

The psychiatrist put down his pen and looked at Chuck. "Dr. Sweigard, I'll make a deal with you. We have a consulting psychiatrist from Standford, Dr. Peter Rosenbaum, who comes here once a month. He should be here in three or four days. He will talk to you and test you anyway he pleases. If he says all of us who have talked to you are wrong . . ."

Chuck interrupted, "All but Dr. Hill."

"Agreed. He is why I don't just proceed with

treatment. I have it on good authority that Dr. Hill is an excellent man. If Rosenbaum agrees with him, fine. If not, if Rosenbaum says that you are psychotic, then you are going to cooperate, or I am going to take whatever steps necessary to treat you as I believe you should be treated. In this case, I'm the doctor. Until then, we'll leave matters up in the air."

PART III

SUMMARY OF PSYCHIATRIC TREATMENT:

. . . He (Sweigard) was presented on two occasions, a month apart to Dr. Peter Rosenbaum, Psychiatric Consultant from Standford University. He was given a series of psychological tests . . . He was actually kept off medication after his first consultant interview.

11 Aug 66
MODESTO

Chuck liked Dr. Rosenbaum after he'd talked with him for only five minutes. The psychiatrist gave two impressions. One, he wasn't trying to prove anything, and two, he wasn't trying to sell anything. After the pleasantries were over, the psychiatrist got down to business.

"Dr. Sweigard, we have to establish a couple of

things first or we are not going to get anywhere. First, I have an open mind. I have read a letter from Dr. Hill that is in your file in which he points out that you have been misdiagnosed because in his words, "... careful review of his Langley Porter records indicate no thought disorders or other signs of a psychosis.' I have looked over the same records and at the moment, I'm inclined to agree with him.

"Now, Dr. Sweigard, I'm going to come at you with as open a mind as I can manage. In return, I want from you the same kind of honesty. No tricks. Try to forget, or at least not to use, what you have been taught about psychiatry. Your knowledge will get in our way. Will you try to be honest?"

Chuck felt a sense of relief. This man was an answer to his prayers. "I certainly will."

"Good. How much medication have you had?"

"Half of what has been prescribed. I've learned how to palm the pills. Most of the time they don't go into my mouth."

"Good. You seem rather alert for a man taking your supposed dosage." He spread a test out on the table between them, right side up to Chuck. "These are questions you probably haven't seen before. This is a new test that hasn't yet been published. Let's start with question number one."

Three hours went by before Rosenbaum was finished. When he was done he put his papers back into his brief case, closed it and looked at Chuck. "I'm in agreement with Hill. There is no psychosis that I can find, not on the basis of this test. I will be back in a month and we will try again. If the results are the same, I'll get you out of here."

"Thank you, doctor, although a thank you is inadequate. Can you put an end to the medication?"

"Let it come from me. Don't say anything against it to your doctor. We could wind up with a professional jealousy problem that none of us want. Go on back to your room, and I'll find your doctor."

He didn't find Chuck's doctor; the young psychiatrist was not in at that particular time, but Dr. Rosenbaum did find the head nurse. "Nurse, Dr. Sweigard's doctor is out at the moment?"

"Yes, sir."

"I'm going to leave him a note. It is my opinion that Dr. Sweigard should have no more medication, that he should go home on weekends, and that he should be given a job of some kind around here. Before writing my diagnosis of this case, I will see the patient once more next month. I would advise no further treatment until after my second visit."

The nurse handed him a pen and a piece of paper. "Please put it in writing."

"Of course."

PART IV

SUMMARY OF PSYCHIATRIC TREATMENT: . . . He was given a series of psychological tests and partook of psychology group discussions. He also was assigned to one of the dining rooms, where he worked efficiently . . .

16 Aug 66
MODESTO

It was just before Tuesday's lunch; the doors that would admit the patients to the noon meal would soon be opened. Chuck admired his handy work, everything was in the proper container on the steam tables and was being kept hot. The service was cafeteria style with two parallel lines. The help passed the loaded dishes across to the patients as they moved their trays. The lines outside the dining room had formed with people waiting for lunch. Who had anything else to do better than wait in line? The clock pointed to noon and the doors were opened.

A woman, the fourth patient in the line on the right picked up her tray in such a manner that she caught Chuck's eye. She had a look on her face that made it look blank, but made it look blank for the wrong reason. Chuck got the feeling that if she relaxed, her face wouldn't be blank. In a moment it wasn't.

She was handed a bowl of hot soup by an attendant who was helping her put it on her tray, and therefore leaning toward her. With a quick movement the patient picked up the bowl of soup and threw it into the face of the woman waiting on her. It was hot and caused a pain-stricken scream.

The thing that hit Chuck was the change on the face of the patient, a look that went from deliberately blank to malevolent glee. He remembered the remark that came from Pastor Jones, "This is Satan's domain."

They helped the burned woman to a different part of the hospital. Chuck went to the back of the kitchen and picked up a mop and a rag. He had the mess cleaned up promptly, but he'd lost his appetite for his own meal. When he'd put the mop back, he kept on walking out through the back door and out on to the grounds. He had the right to do that now. Since Dr. Rosenbaum's visit the restrictions on him had been few, and he had every other week end at home. That was a mixed blessing, Cathy was as cold as ice, and the children, as per instructions, kept their distance. In some ways, home was lonelier than the hospital.

The yard maintenance crew members were eating their lunches under one of the trees, taking advantage of the shade. A member of the ground crew who noticed him put his lunch down and walked over in such a way that his path would intercept Chuck's. When he was close he took off his hat and spoke.

"Dr. Sweigard."

Chuck was surprised. "Do I know you?"

"No, sir, but I know you. You treated my granddaughter. She had something wrong with her throat. We'd taken her to a couple of doctors without any result, but you fixed her up."

"What was her name?" The gardener told him. "Oh, yes, I remember her."

He did remember her; it had been an unusual

case. The trouble in swallowing had not been physical but psychosomatic, and Chuck had gotten to the root of the matter, leaving the family thinking it had been physical, but talking to them indirectly about the real problem.

"You work here, I gather?"

"Yes, sir, I'm the chief gardener, but that isn't what I wanted to talk about. We're Christians, and we know about you, and we know you're not crazy. We've been told that you're in here because of your faith, and we believe it. I just wanted you to know that all of us, our whole church prays for you every day, and our pastor prays for you every Sunday. We want God to get you out of here so you can have peace and go back to healing people."

It was totally unexpected and it hit Chuck right where he hurt. With his eyes swimming in tears he said, "Thank you very much."

He walked away. No grown man likes to be seen crying.

Back in the hospital and in control of himself, he surveyed the bulletin board. There was an announcement that he hadn't noticed before, a notice that the hospital chaplain held a Sunday morning service at ten a.m. for Protestants, and that Father Joseph from the local Catholic Parish came at one thirty p.m. to hold mass.

The name of the hospital chaplain was obviously a feminine name, and Chuck wondered what she was like. He walked toward the administrative part of the hospital and found the chaplain's office. Her door was open and she was in, she had just finished eating her lunch at her desk, and she was picking up the scraps and getting them into the waste basket. Chuck figured she was a brown bagger because of a weight problem. She looked like she had to struggle with it and he knew by personal experience that the temptations to overeat were fewer at a desk than in a cafeteria or a restaurant.

She was mildly interested in him as a patient. The interest quickened when she found that he was a doctor-patient. That was unusual. She asked him a little about himself, and was rewarded when Chuck asked her questions about herself. She was the first woman chaplain and she was the first woman graduate of Union Theological Seminary in New York to be ordained by the Methodist Church. This should have been a whole series of red flags to Chuck, but it wasn't. He was new to the things of the Lord and to him a seminary was a seminary, and all Christians were believers.

She looked up from Chuck to the door. A man was waiting to see her. She explained to Chuck that she had appointments for the afternoon, but she'd love to continue her conversation with him. Would he be coming to the Sunday service? He said he would; it was not his weekend to go home. They agreed that after the service, they'd go to the hospital coffee shop and have a cup together. They would be able to continue their conversation then.

Sunday morning Chuck was seated in the chapel a little before ten. The audience was "rag, tag, and bob-tailed." He smiled when he reminded himself that he was one who was present from the real nut ward.

The chaplain came in and assumed command.

She announced that it would be a simple service
and then she opened it with a word of prayer. After
the "amen" she wanted to know if anyone had a
hymn they would like to sing. Someone gave her a
number and everyone opened their hymnals to turn
to it. The singing would have been ragged, but the
woman at the piano was good, and she kept the
group together and helped them keep time. Chuck
lifted his voice in song for the first time in many
months and sang the words by J. H. Sammis.
"When we walk with the Lord in the light of His
Word, What a glory He sheds on our way! While
we do His good will, He abides with us still, and
with all who will trust and obey. Trust and obey,
for there's no other way, To be happy in Jesus, But
to trust and obey."

The first verse was all that Chuck could sing, he
was afraid he'd choke up, but it was a blessing. He
was blessed right down to his shoes. It was as
though the hymn had been written for Chuck Sweigard. it made the chapel worthwhile. The sermon
didn't. It was a little homily that could best be described as innocuous. No one would learn anything, but then no one would be upset either. Chuck
didn't hold the matter against the chaplain, she had
her problems. There could be things easily said that
would trigger a bad reaction in some member of
that rather peculiar audience. She would have to be
innocuous.

When the service was over, she and Chuck went
to the coffee shop. They sat at a small table, drank
coffee, and Chuck talked. He was not wise to the
ways of the religious world and he didn't know

enough to check someone out before he unloaded. He thought he was talking to a chaplain, and therefore someone who was a Christian by Chuck's definition, so he unloaded his experiences, his feelings and his struggles. She interrupted only occasionally, and then only to ask a question.

When Chuck was through, she gave him counsel. "It may be, Dr. Sweigard, that you're basing your experiences on the wrong thing. The business of the belief in the deity of Jesus is rather a thing of the past, or something that the uneducated and uninformed still cling to. There are many great scholars of the Bible and of Christian history who believe that the concept of the deity of Christ, so called, developed over a period of centuries until it got to its almost universal acceptance during the middle ages. Many of us who have studied professionally are quite convinced that Jesus was really the illegitimate son of Mary and a Roman soldier."

She was going to go on with the matter, but she noticed that all the color had drained out of Chuck's face. He was stunned. He had had experiences with the risen Christ, had had some touch of His glory, His power, and His Holiness. He had found his own sins forgiven by the glorified Son of God, and to hear Him referred to as the bastard son of a Roman soldier, left Chuck feeling like he was going to vomit.

The chaplain was apologetic. "I'm sorry, I didn't mean to upset you so much, you seemed like an intelligent man who would be interested in the facts of the matter."

Chuck was stuck. What could he say? Of what

value would a testimony be, if it came from someone who had been declared legally insane? Suddenly feeling older and wiser, he got up and walked
away without saying anything further. He said
something to himself. "Pastor Jones, you were oh,
so, right."

PART V

22 Sept 66
MODESTO

More than a month rolled around before Dr.
Rosenbaum was back in Modesto. It was more like
six weeks. But he finally came. He and Chuck were
using the office of the resident psychiatrist, sitting
as they had sat six weeks before. The window was
still in place, so were the bars. Chuck had learned to
hate them. Rosenbaum opened the conversation by
talking about medicine in general and then about
pediatrics in particular. Finally he paused.

"Dr. Sweigard, we are back to square one.
Every time I ask you a question, I can see you hesi-
tate and think, 'What is the psychiatric significance
of that question?' and then you scramble back into
what you know about psychiatry—which is getting
to be more and more, incidentally—and try to figure out how you should answer. We will get nowhere at all if you keep that up.

"I really do have your best interests at heart;
you are my patient. Furthermore, I am quite con-

vinced that you are not psychotic and my questions are now being asked with that in mind. I want to talk to you about medicine because I can find out a great deal about a man when I ask him about his work. So, please, just answer my questions in an open and honest way, will you?"

A little ashamed, Chuck answered, "I'll try."

"Good. Now, why did you leave the Medical Group?"

"I was fired."

"That's simple and straightforward. Why did they fire you?"

"Their reasons or mine?"

"Yours."

"I think that my psychiatric record was a source of embarrassment to them. Worse, they didn't want a doctor in the Group who witnessed and prayed with his patients." Chuck answered that with fear and trembling. It was perilously close to paranoia.

"And so you went into practice for yourself. How do you think you differ from other pediatricians?"

"Besides religious differences?"

"Yes."

Chuck began to talk about his approach to the whole person. As he talked his enthusiasm increased. Rosenbaum would interject questions, good ones that kept Chuck on the track. They talked for an hour before the psychiatrist held up his hand and stood up. "Let's go outside for a bit."

Chuck readily agreed, he hated the inside under any circumstances. Together they walked across the green lawn toward an empty bench near a tree, but in the sun. It was not a warm day and the sunshine would feel good. As soon as they were seated, Rosenbaum started talking.

"It is good that we come out here. In an office, one never knows who's listening, and I want to say some things to you in a confidential way.

"I, too, like my work, Dr. Sweigard. I like to come here once a month and help. If I were to write to the staff here, what I really think about your case and what has been done to you, they might get so angry that I would not be asked back. So, I am going to write a very polite letter, if I can, saying you are not psychotic and giving very good reasons. I will try not to be too angry in the letter. But, I am angry. I'm going to talk to them in a different way than I write. You are a religious zealot. People who do not know a religious zealot when they see one should not try to practice psychiatry."

Chuck felt his stomach muscles begin to relax. The light at the end of the tunnel could be easily seen. Rosenbaum continued.

"I do not mean by what I'm saying that you have no problems, we all have problems and you've got some big ones. They showed up a little in college, they showed up a little more in medical school and they came to a head in your marriage. Your conversion has helped you and hurt your wife. Neither one of you are out of the woods, but you are not psychotic."

Chuck spoke up. "We have a belief in sanctification that it is a gradual and continuing . . ."

Rosenbaum held up his hand for silence.

"Please, doctor, don't try to testify to me. I know quite a little about your religion, even about Pentecostals. Let me continue. You need help. Go see Hill, he is a good man, and if you go with your wife, he may be able to help her. She wasn't all-together either, and your conversion has been more than she can handle. Also, I would advise medication. You have a drive toward perfection both in yourself and in your practice and you have very bad tensions at home. You can get yourself wound up again to where they will put you back inside here once more. Whatever tranquilizer they recommend, take it. If you don't like it, try another, but until your tensions inside and out are decreased, keep giving yourself a little sedation."

Dr. Rosenbaum got up. "Now we'll go back inside and I will write my letter and try to be calm. Then I will talk to them and blow my top. You won't be in here very much longer."

Chuck stuck out his hand and Dr. Rosenbaum shook it as Chuck spoke to him. "Thank you very, very much, Doctor." He started to add something about this being an answer to many prayers but realized that that would be resented. He was learning. Sometimes you say something and sometimes you don't.

PART VI

22 Sept 66 cont.

Because of his time with Dr. Rosenbaum, Chuck had been relieved of his duties in the dining room for the day, so he stood in line to go to lunch. His line was parallel to the line that was using the other steam table. There was a young man in his early twenties, obviously of Mexican descent who was even with Chuck in the other line. The young man tried to strike up a friendly conversation with the man ahead of him and the man behind him and got nowhere with either. Chuck watched him and as he came off his line with his tray in his hands, Chuck with his tray followed him, and sat at the same table, across from him.

"My name is Chuck."

"I'm Tony Hernandez."

"And you're a Christian."

He looked up from his soup, startled. "How did you know?"

"The Lord let me know. Why are you here?"

Tony was eager to tell his story. He had gone to a meeting Sunday night with a Protestant friend. Tony and his family were Catholic. The meeting had been interesting, and the man who preached had talked about Jesus and the forgiveness of sins.

"I know the words," Tony said. "I've heard most of them all my life, but this was different. Jesus wasn't a dying figure on a cross. He was a living Savior and Lord. At the end of the meeting, I went forward and accepted Christ. When I got home, I told my parents. They were upset."

"I'll bet they were."

"Anyway, I went into my bedroom and got down on my knees, and for the first time in my life I did it because I really wanted to, and I started to pray and to praise the Lord. Then I don't know why, but it changed, and it wasn't English or Spanish anymore, and it got louder and louder. I was having a wonderful time, feeling better and happier than I have ever felt in my life. My parents, they didn't understand. They thought something had snapped up here." He pointed to his head. "They called an ambulance, and they brought me to this place. How do I get out?"

"It's not always easy," Chuck admitted ruefully, "But in your case the Lord has a message for you. You will not be here long."

Tony looked at him in a peculiar way. "I don't know why I believe you, but I do."

"You should, Tony, the message is from the Lord."

In a few days they would both be out, but Chuck would be out only temporarily.

CHAPTER EIGHT

PART I

24 Nov 66
MODESTO

Six weeks had gone by since Chuck's release from his Modesto incarceration. It had been a pointless interruption in a hopeless situation. Chuck gradually worked his way right back into what he had endured before they had carted him away. His practice was in the same place, with many of the same patients who drifted back as they heard of his return. There were the same peculiar looks from the same kind of people who wondered a bit about a doctor who had been in a couple of insane asylums. Home was the same only worse. Cathy was growing increasingly frustrated as her influence over Chuck continued to be non-existent.

From her point of view, there was also the problem of the children. It had been easy enough to say that their father was crazy, and that he would return to being his old nasty self in due time. But that hadn't worked out as planned. Cathy and Chuck had increasingly bitter arguments from time to time, but Chuck was fighting the tendency with all his heart and with all his prayers. The children were growing more aware of his efforts and Chuck was being very careful in front of them not to answer back if he could help it. They were beginning to have mixed emotions.

It is natural for a child to want fellowship with a father, and the children were seeing him sometimes when he was at his best. That was frightening to Cathy. The wall that she had put up between them was harder and harder to keep in place. It was easy when Chuck was institutionalized. Then there was no evidence for anything contrary to what she wanted to teach them, namely that their father's view of God and the world was a crazy view; that's why he was in an asylum. Case closed. But when Chuck was home—gentle, considerate and friendly to his sons and daughters, the story and the perspective began to be questioned. The only way she could continue her charade was to keep Chuck off balance with remarks that would upset him. She was good at it, and home was not a pleasant place.

From Chuck's point of view, it was not as malicious as it seemed. He could remember how he felt before he knew the Lord and had had the experiences that had convinced him. He would have given short shrift to anyone who had told him to plan his life on the basis that Christ might return any day and judge the world, that this Jesus of Nazareth should be the Lord of every man's life every hour he lived, that life in this world is transient and comparatively unimportant and that personal ambition is ungodly. If someone had tried to sell that to him a few years ago he'd have died laughing. He could see more and more clearly just how poorly those who really were committed to Christ fit into this world.

He could see Cathy's point of view because it had been his. She had been innoculated against the truth by religious teaching, a liberal teaching that taught that man was basically good. A Biblical view of man that placed all men justly in sin and under condemnation apart from Christ was anathema to her. This in spite of the Episcopalian liturgy which she spoke unthinkingly almost every Sunday, but never really heard.

While Chuck had been safely confined at Modesto, she had gone on a trip to see her scientist brother about Chuck and about her relationship with him. She had taken some of the notes that Chuck had written to himself as he had been thinking through his own faith. The statements contained in those notes, that all men were born in sin, that all men were basically evil, that all men had to be redeemed by the blood of Christ; all of this added up to insanity as far as her brother was concerned and he told Cathy to pack up and go back to Pennsylvania. Her father and mother would be glad to have her and their grandchildren back. Why should she stay with someone who was crazy?

She had Chuck in a three-way bind. His practice was marginal. There was no communication on any real level at home. (There is no fellowship between light and darkness.) Third, and distressing to Chuck, she had no communication with Dr. Hill. Nor did he. He was still driving up to Stockton to see the psychiatrist on a professional basis, but he was going alone. Cathy had stopped making the trip. She did not want to confuse the issue with her "minor" problems, when the major problem was Chuck and his insanity. Chuck's problems weren't being solved either.

PART II

16 Dec 66
STOCKTON

Dr. Hill was a thoroughly professional, well trained and knowledgeable psychiatrist, but he was having trouble with Chuck. During their usual Friday afternoon session in mid-December he told him so.

"Chuck, you're not cooperating."

They were in his downtown office not far from the hospital. Too close to the hospital as far as Chuck was concerned. He liked to stay far away from there. The two men had a certain affection for each other, and certainly mutual respect, but there was a battle going on nonetheless.

Chuck returned the question. "What is there to cooperate about?" There was no answer for a minute and Chuck continued. "What was the diagnosis from Langley Porter?"

"I'd rather not say."

"Come on, what's the good of hiding it?"

"All right, it was 'Paranoid reaction, paranoid state.' "

"That's a big step down from Winkler's diagnosis at Stockton, isn't it? I happen to know what he said, 'Schizophrenic Reaction—Paranoid Type.' "

"That's true. It's a step down."

"You don't, and you haven't agreed with either one of them, have you? I know that you have written that you do not believe me to be psychotic, but what exactly do you think?"

"I'm not sure it is wise to say."

"Come on. You're not dealing with a child nor an ignorant layman. You know what I know, but what do you think?"

"I would say that your episode was a Psychoneurotic Dissociative Reaction as characterized by temporary feelings of disassociation."

"And what do you mean by that?"

"To put it simply, you are on this planet and you can function on it, but you're not one of us. Furthermore, I don't think you want to be one of us, and this treatment or attempted treatment is getting to be pointless. I'm not getting anywhere with you."

Chuck thought hard for a minute. Was he walking back into the same trap? Was he talking to someone in a way that they could not understand? Was he going to make himself look worse again? He decided to take the risk and speak his mind.

"I'm afraid of complicating things and I say this with a tight stomach, but I'll try to explain. Jesus said to His disciples, 'You are in this world, but not of it.' That is what you have just said to me. If you make me 'well' from your point of view, won't you put me back to where I was when I wanted to commit suicide? Do you want me to return to that?"

"No, I don't, but before we go on with that line of thought, I have another question for you. There are other people who share, or say they share your beliefs. They too believe that Jesus of Nazereth was God incarnate, but they are not my patients, and they seem to get along rather well in what I would call a normal world. How do you explain that?"

Chuck got up out of his chair and walked over to the office window. When he looked out he could see the street which the ambulance had used when it took him to the State Hospital the first time. He hated the possibility of ever making that trip again. That feeling made him want to shut his mouth or lie, but his conscience was nudging him. Dr. Hill, too, was someone for whom Christ had died. Chuck had to talk, but he was going to do it with great care.

"I think that the difference lies in two different areas. There is a sense in which some people in our culture are Christian in the same way that there are others in other cultures who are Buddhists. That's what they were born into, and that is the way they were raised. If you asked these Christians raised in a Christian environment if they believed in the deity of Christ, they would probably say that they did, but saying it would cost them nothing. There is no committal. That's where I was. It is hard for me to be sure, but I think that when I was 'normal' and in church the Sunday before I tried to commit suicide, if you had asked me if I believed in Christ, I think I would have said yes.

"Now I'm not trying to argue that every person

who calls himself a Christian and is 'normal' is an uncommitted Christian. Are there some normal people who are really committed to Christ? I don't know. If there are and if they fit into this world too well, all I can say is that either they are lying, or that God has not dealt with them as He has dealt with me. I'm not objecting, that is His prerogative."

Hill pursed his lips for a moment. "That was a mouthful. Let me ask you this, you don't want to be like those who really 'fit in' do you?"

"Sometimes I want to very badly."

"Why don't you?"

"I know too much and I've experienced too much. I can't go back."

Dr. Hill got up out of his chair and walked over to the window. He stood beside Chuck. "I have to tell you two things. First, you are not psychotic and don't let anyone talk you into thinking so. You are capable of practicing medicine and you should do so. The second thing is this. Until you want to be part of us, to see things as the rest of us see them, I can't really do anything for you, and we're wasting time and money."

"Not exactly, Dr. Hill. I can't practice the medicine that you say I'm capable of practicing unless I'm under your care."

"I am aware of that. I will leave you listed as a patient, and will see you occasionally, but I want your word that you will try to find someone else."

"I promise." Chuck smiled, "One more thing. I like your beard; would you mind if I tried to copy it."

Hill returned the smile. "Help yourself."

PART III

20 Dec 66
MODESTO

At the dinner table, Cathy made a tart observation. "You didn't shave this morning. Are you trying to look like one of your high class patient's parents?"

"No, I'm growing a beard. I want to see how it looks."

"On you it will look terrible."

"It doesn't look bad on Dr. Hill."

"Dr. Hill my left foot. You want to look like Jesus. You're still as kooky as ever. You have no decent practice, you're not making enough money to even buy a decent car, and you spend your time hanging around with a bunch of Pentecostals who are as crazy as you are. Now go upstairs and shave."

Chuck got up, but walked toward the front door.

"Where are you going?"

"Where I'll feel at home."

She watched him leave by the front door, and then she went to the window to be sure he drove away. Once the tail lights of his car had disappeared, she went to the phone. When someone said hello she asked if the doctor was there.

He came to the phone. "Yes." It was a very non-committal yes.

"This is Cathy Sweigard."

His voice suddenly increased in warmth. "Yes,

Cathy, nice to hear your voice. Is something wrong?"

"Yes. He's gone to be with those Pentecostal people again. It's really terrible. After he's been with them for a while, no one can do anything with him. It's as though he's not even in this world."

"This might be a good time to talk to him, I just phoned Frank and he's not on call tonight. I'll call Jeff and see if he can get away. The three of us have been praying for your husband at the meetings of the Christian Medical Society. We've made your husband's condition a matter of daily prayer between us. If we are all three free, we'll come over. Maybe we can pray with him and talk to him. If we're not coming I'll call you right back and let you know.

"Thank you, doctor." She hung up the phone for a moment and then made another call.

When the phone was answered she identified herself. "Marj, this is Cathy Sweigard. Is my husband's car parked across the street in front of Jim's house?"

"Just a minute, I'll go look."

When she returned to the phone, she had the news Cathy wanted. "Your husband just pulled up and parked."

"Thank you."

Chuck got out of his car and walked up to the door, rang the bell and waited for a few seconds. The tall, young milkman greeted him warmly. "Come in, we're having coffee."

"Thank you." Inside the house, Chuck looked

around at the mess. There wasn't anything in the home that was in its proper place. There was no semblance of neatness, but there was no hate either. A couple of other men from the Pentecostal fellowship had dropped in to talk to Jim and they all were happy to greet the doctor.

"Problems, Dr. Chuck?" Jim pointed to a chair. "Sit over here."

"Thank you. No, no new problems, it just gets so bad at home that I have to get out of there. It's good to be where I'm with brothers."

Jim spoke soberly. "You're always welcome here." The other two men expressed similar offers of hospitality and then they picked up the conversation they'd been having when Chuck came. They had been talking about some of the growing problems in their fellowship. It was beginning to come apart at the seams. Chuck listened for a while and then decided he didn't want to listen to that mess either, and he interrupted.

"Excuse me for butting in, but would you three fellows pray for me and lay your hands on me?"

"Sure." Jim pointed to a comparatively clear spot in the middle of the living room floor and said, "Why don't you kneel right there."

Chuck did, and with his hands folded in front of him and his eyes closed he knelt and waited. The three men put their hands on him and all three began to pray at once, quietly but with strong emotional feeling in their voices. Chuck felt himself relax and began to experience an inner peace. He opened his mouth and joined in. He was sure he wasn't praying in English. It was a very short prayer. The phone rang. It jarred the room into silence.

Jim picked it up. "Hello." There was a moment while he listened. "Just a minute." He looked at Chuck, "It's your wife."

"How would she know I'm here?"

"I think I know. I think the woman who lives across the street, Marj, is a friend of Marie, your secretary. That probably makes her a friend of your wife, and I think that Marj would tell anything to anybody."

Chuck took the phone from Jim. "Yes."

"You get your ass out of there and bring it home right now." The receiver was slammed into place.

Chuck turned to Jim. "I've got to go home."

"Dr. Chuck, why do you always do what she says; you're the man in the house?"

"Since you've prayed for me I feel different, and I think that when I get home, I'll point that out. But, I'll point it out gently. I don't think our marriage is going to last very much longer, but I want it to last as long as possible. I don't think divorce is pleasing to the Lord. The other thing is, that I want to be sure in my own heart that I did all I could to keep things together."

Jim shrugged. "I guess that's the right attitude. God bless you brother, and we'll be praying for you."

Chuck looked around and suddenly realized there were only men present. "Where are your wives?" He looked at all three men. One of them, whom Chuck didn't remember seeing before that evening answered.

"They're having their own prayer meeting. They are over at my house. We'll call them right now and tell them to start praying for you too."

"Thank you." Chuck took his leave.

He parked in his driveway and walked into the house. The alcove behind the front door opened directly into the living room. There were three doctors sitting there, two on the couch and one in an easy chair. They got to their feet as Chuck came into the room.

Chuck knew all three of them. One was an orthopedic surgeon. He was, many years later, to ask Chuck's forgiveness for what he was doing this night. A second was a general practitioner and the third a general surgeon. Besides being M.D.s, the three had other things in common. They were members of the Christian Medical Society. They were Fundamentalists. They all suspected that all Pentecostals were at least a little bit crazy. They knew very little about psychiatry.

Chuck turned to Cathy and with a firmness and a courage that owed its existence in part to the prayer meeting he'd just left, he asked her a pointed question.

"When are you going to stop parading our problems before the public in general and the Medical profession in particular? The differences we have are our business and none of theirs."

Cathy blanched and the surgeon quickly spoke.

"Look, Chuck, no one is angry with you, we're just here to try to help."

"Who needs help?" There was a long and awkward pause. "Did you three come in one car?"

It was the surgeon who spoke again. "Yes, we came in my car."

"Where is it?"

"It's parked down the street."

"In the dark?"

"Yes. We thought if you saw our cars you wouldn't come in."

"Why do you say 'we'? Why don't you tell the truth? Cathy thought I might not come in and she told you to park in the dark and you did what Cathy told you to do. Don't feel too badly, an awful lot of men do. Now let me tell you something doctor. You parked in the dark because it isn't the Lord who sent you."

"Now, now, Chuck, listen to reason." The irony of the situation was that the surgeon was on his way to his divorce also, but didn't know it yet. "Why would someone who was . . ." He hesitated a minute trying to find a diplomatic way of wording what he wanted to say. He started over. "Why would someone who was feeling well want to grow a beard to look like Christ?"

"What makes you think that? If you keep on believing everything you're told without checking into it, you're going to kill some patients. I started a beard to see if it would be becoming. If it is a sign of insanity, I'll be glad to shave it off."

Everyone was still standing, no one had resumed their seat and the tension in the room was palpable. The surgeon tried again.

"We hear you have plans for traveling around, 'sowing the Word'."

"She told you that too, did she? It's hard for me to remember that everything I tell my wife is going to be broadcast throughout the medical community. Yes, I have hope of entering some form of the ministry."

"If you were to be a minister wouldn't God have sent you to seminary instead of medical school?"

"Weren't you a missionary?"

"Yes, for several years."

"Didn't you have to go to Bible school?"

"Yes."

"If you were a missionary and became a full-time practicing doctor and have remained sane, how does it happen that if I'm a doctor who becomes some kind of a missionary, I'm insane?"

The orthopedic surgeon spoke up in a quiet and steady voice. "I think we're avoiding the point. Chuck, those who know you best, your wife, your secretary, and those of us who can see the tension under which you are laboring are worried about you. You are overdoing. I don't think there can be much argument about that."

Chuck knew that there could be argument about that, but the argument would be pointless. How could a man live in the constant contention in which he lived and not look like he was overdoing it? There was no reason to try to protest, and the orthopedic surgeon seemed to have a decent attitude. Chuck let him continue.

"Is it so wrong to ask you to go back to the hospital and put yourself under care for a few days or a few weeks until you've calmed down again? It would seem to be the wisest course."

"It seems good to you because you don't know what it's like. You're asking me in a casual and friendly way to go back to hell. The answer would be absolutely no, but I know the alternative. You call the big boys in white and I get taken. I don't stand a chance in a trial. Once a thief, always a thief; once crazy, always crazy. With three M.D.s and a determined wife against me, I'm going to be in there one way or another, sooner or later." He paused for a moment and thought before he continued. "This is Tuesday the 20th of December. I can get my office in order by Thursday night or Friday morning. I'll turn myself into Stockton on the 23rd. Now you three sneak on back down to where Cathy told you to park your car, and get out of here."

They left feeling slightly used.

PART IV

STOCKTON STATE HOSPITAL
510 East Magnolia St.
Stockton, California 95202

RT-3

RELEASE SUMMARY
NAME: SWEIGARD, Charles (MI)
No: #104301
FILE SECTION I—E

PRESENT ILLNESS: Dr. Sweigard's present admission occurred after a period of private treatment with Dr. Hill in Stockton. Differences between his wife were becoming so great and each was becoming so agitated that it was thought advisable he enter the hospital. He was clear and cooperative in being here but spoke about his feelings about religion and experience of conversion as if it was very real to him. He showed considerable denial of the reality of his medical practice, of the fact that he was financially insolvent, and of the fact that he and his wife had major differences of opinion. His affect was not appropriate in view of these realistic situations and was suggestive of hypermanic attitude. While he has been in the hospital Dr. Sweigard has been entirely cooperative. He has taken the attitude that it is best not to belabor others with his religious feelings. On the other hand he has been extremely busy in the activities on the ward and reading medical literature. He did not tolerate Stelazine but has made a good response to Elavil, 25mgm., t.i.d. He says that he has not felt in such good spirits for a long time. Conversations with his wife indicate that there are very large differences between them and it is evident that divorce is being considered. This subject does not upset Dr. Sweigard at the present moment. He is very intent upon *retaining his medical license...*

18 Jan 67 NOTE: DISCHARGE TREATMENT COMPLETED, CONDITION IMPROVED. APPROVED, ISSUE CERTIFICATE OF COMPETENCE. FINAL DIAGNOSIS: MANIC DEPRESSIVE REACTION, MANIC TYPE.

The Chuck Sweigard who checked himself into the Stockton State Hospital on the twenty-third of December was altogether different than the Chuck Sweigard who had been taken to Stockton in an ambulance in August of 1965. The first entrance had found him surrounded by blissful ignorance. Not so this time. He walked in knowing what the psychiatrist was going to want to hear, and he had figured out how to say it without in any way denying his own faith. His knowledge of psychiatry had been greatly enhanced.

His psychiatrist was a young resident who had just started his professional career at Stockton. Chuck could lead him where he wanted him to go. The first trick was to not let himself get too heavily doped, so when he was given Stelazine he knew that it was too tough and he'd want to stay off it. Fighting that drug, he might not be able to keep control of the situation.

It was easy to get off it. Chuck knew what to do and when to do it. The psychiatrist bought his act and put Chuck on an easier drug, Elavil. The dosage was supposed to be t.i.d., three times a day, but Chuck palmed the first two of the day and took the third when he was going to be going to sleep anyway.

During his sessions with the psychiatrist, he gave enough information to make his agitation plausible, but not enough to lead to committal. Chuck lost his agitation anyway whenever he got far enough away from Cathy. The young psychiatrist congratulated himself on the handling of Chuck's case, and signed a release in less than a month. Something should be said on his behalf. He knew Chuck was not psychotic. He didn't make the same mistake that some of his "betters" did.

PART V

19 Jan 67
MODESTO

It was Thursday and Chuck was back in his office. He was trying to get things in shape so that he could start practicing the following Monday. He'd get some of his old patients back, and slowly, some new ones. Word would get around that he was working again, and he'd get the rejects, but he'd get a few paying patients too. It was in God's hands.

Things were no better at home. Cathy was once again bitterly disappointed. Her husband had gone to the hospital but he hadn't been "cured." He was still willing to practice medicine for nothing. The ambitious, driving doctor that she had married was gone and she didn't seem to be able to get him back.

Had there been any other hope, any hope of another marriage, any hope of money from any other source, she would have been long gone. As it was she felt trapped.

She had married Chuck Sweigard on one basis and on one picture of what life was to be like, and it hadn't turned out right at all. She hated housework, she hated out-of-style clothes, and she hated old cars. Her one hope was to get her husband back on track, and her hopes of doing this were fading. He was stubborn about his illness and he was going to stay that way. She had pretty well made up her mind to leave and she was waiting for the right time to have the final show down, and take off. She couldn't leave for a little while. There wasn't enough money in the bank account to buy tickets. That would take a little more time.

PART VI

12 Feb 67
MODESTO

She started to broach the subject. It was a Sunday evening and she had taken her usual place in bed with a book. Chuck came in about ten p.m. She opened the conversation and prepared for battle.

"How are all your nutty Pentecostal friends?"

"I haven't been with them." Chuck got a hanger out of the closet and began to undress.

"That's new and different, where have you been this time?"

"I went with Bob Elliot to the First Presbyterian Church. Bob is still practicing pediatrics at the Medical Group, and they got a flyer on a new psychiatric group in Sacramento under a Dr. Harris. One of Harris' psychiatrists came to the First Presbyterian Church to talk tonight on family problems, particularly marriage relationships. He presented Harris' approach to therapy. He had some good stuff and he presented it well. Bob and I talked to him after the meeting, and he agreed to take me off Dr. Hill's hands if I'd attend one of their once a week therapy sessions in Sacramento."

Cathy was more than molified—she was hopeful. Maybe she'd give it one more try. "Sounds good."

"There is a catch."

"Oh?" Suspicion in her voice again.

"They prefer couples. They would like you to come too."

"What'll we do with the kids?"

"Bob volunteered the services of his wife as a Friday afternoon baby-sitter."

"All right, I'll go, but if this or something like it doesn't work pretty soon, the children and I are going back to Pennsylvania. I've just about had it."

Chuck hung his suit in the closet and sat on the end of the bed in his underwear holding his pajamas in one hand. He looked Cathy straight in the eye. "I can't make you stay if you decide to go, but it is going to be your decision. I will do all in my power to get along with you. God has put a love in my heart for you and the children, and if you do leave, you'll have to answer to Him."

"You won't do all in your power. You won't go back to a successful medical practice and forget your Pentecostal nuts."

"That's not in my power." He quoted St. Paul and put it in the first person. "I am not my own; I'm bought with a price."

Cathy made an unladylike noise and went back to reading her book.

CHAPTER NINE

PART I

24 Feb 67
SACRAMENTO

Chuck drove east on Howe Street in the northeast part of Sacramento looking for the address. He found it, it was a complex of office buildings where the Harris Group held some of their sessions. He turned right, drove a hundred and fifty feet and turned right again into the parking lot. The buildings were comparatively new, made of adobe brick and almost Moorish in design. They were separated from each other by walks, greenery and fountains. Chuck and Cathy found the right part of the complex and walked up the stairs. Their meeting room was on the second floor.

It was a large room, well carpeted and furnished with comfortable chairs placed in a circle. All but two of the chairs were occupied; the Sweigards were a couple of minutes late. When they sat down all the chairs were filled and the therapist called the session to order.

"We're going to get acquainted today. We're going to use first names. We'll start on my left and go around the circle. Give your first name, tell us a little about yourself and tell us why you are here."

There were four people among the ten who were

going to be important to the Sweigards. First and foremost was the therapist. His work was to be crucial. Then there was a Baptist couple who were sitting opposite Chuck and Cathy. Her name was Jane. Cathy thought of her as Plain Jane. She was with her husband Frank. Jane was by far the dominant of the two, and would do most of the talking, for both of them. She was overweight, a little sloppy in her dress and very outspoken about being a Baptist, and having no intention of having her faith upset by anything that went on in the session. In many ways, she was the opposite of Cathy who was slim, trim, tanned and well-groomed. The two woman took almost an instant dislike to each other and the sparks would soon be flying.

There was a salesman sitting next to Jane who admitted to having considerable trouble trying to live with his third wife. She had left him, but he hoped the separation would be temporary. He readily admitted that the problem was his. He got angry easily and often.

In a few minutes it was Chuck's turn. He was a much wiser Chuck than he had been three years before. He told of his experience in the kitchen, of his conversion, of his no longer needing glasses, of other habits that had cleared up. Then he told of his vision, of seeing history from the cross. Trying very hard not to be dishonest he told the story trying to play down the supernatural aspects of the experience. He made the story quite believable by a quiet and calm presentation. He was very careful to not try to convince anyone of anything by the way he spoke. It was a take-it-or-leave-it story told in a friendly manner.

Jane never took her eyes off him. She was fascinated. "That is the most wonderful thing I've heard in years. Why did they put you in an institution?" Chuck smiled and ducked the question. "That's what we're here to find out."

Then it was Cathy's turn. "I'm Cathy, and I'm here to try to help my husband, who has been sick."

The salesman wanted to know more. "What kind of sick?"

"To put it bluntly," Cathy answered, "he was declared incompetent by the State of California and found to be psychotic by several psychiatrists."

The therapist, a young M.D., began to look through papers he was holding on his lap. He was not the same psychiatrist who had spoken at the Presbyterian Church in Modesto, but he was similar in many ways. Chuck had the feeling that he was at peace with himself whether for good or for bad reasons, that he was in charge of this situation, and that he was well-trained. He spoke to Cathy.

"Just a minute, Cathy. I have a file on Chuck, and the idea that he is or was psychotic is not universally held. There's a letter from Dr. Hill, whom you know, and who is well thought of in our field. Dr. Hill disagrees with the State's diagnosis and gives good reasons. Then there is a letter from a Standford psychiatrist, a Dr. Rosenbaum. He politely suggests to the State Hospital in Modesto that if they don't know a religious zealot from a psychotic, they ought to get out of the business of psychiatry. The assumption that your husband is or was psychotic is not universally agreed upon and for the purpose of these sessions, it will not be assumed."

Jane took up the cudgel. "Why do you think he was crazy?"

Cathy corrected her, "Is crazy. To start with that dream he told you about he doesn't think it was a dream. He thinks he was wide awake and that God gave him a vision. He believes he actually saw those things."

Jane hadn't gone to Baptist Sunday School for those years for nothing. She could quote the King James. She promptly did. " 'And it shall come to pass in the last days, saith God, I will pour out my spirit upon all flesh; and your sons and your daughters shall prophesy, and your young men shall see visions . . . ' What's the matter with having something happen that's in the Bible and supposed to happen?"

"If the vision identifies you with Jesus Christ?" There was more than a little sarcasm in Cathy's question. This setup was not to her liking and she was getting uncomfortable.

Jane turned to Chuck. "Did you think you were Jesus Christ?"

"No, not at all. I thought I was seeing through the eyes of Jesus what Jesus was seeing when He was on the cross. I have never confused my person with His."

"That's a lie." This from Cathy.

The therapist spoke again. "Just a minute,

Cathy, Dr. Hill states in his letter that he agrees with Chuck. Did Chuck ever say he thought he was Jesus Christ?"

"No, but he said he could see through His eyes. What's the difference?"

"The difference is the difference between sanity and insanity."

The salesman, who had given his name as John, spoke up again. "Cathy, when your husband had this vision, or whatever, did you call a shrink?" He looked at the therapist, "Excuse me, please."

The therapist grinned. "That's all right. I'm used to it."

Cathy answered. "I called two. Neither was available."

"Then whom did you call?"

"A minister friend."

"The Pastor of the church you attend?"

"No, I go to the Episcopal Church."

"Where did you meet this preacher guy you did call?"

"He and Chuck are acquainted, and I've played tennis with him several times. We both played at the racquet club."

The therapist interjected a question. "And between tennis games, you talked to him about Chuck's problems?"

"Of course."

John scratched his head. "Something bothers me. Most doctors I know have friends who are doctors. Didn't your husband have a friend who is a doctor? Why didn't you call another doctor?"

"I called the minister. He knew Chuck too, and he brought a doctor with him when he came to the house."

"What kind of a doctor?"

"An M.D."

John persisted. "What was his practice?"

"Orthopedic surgery."

"What's that got to do with psychiatry? Did your husband practice alone?"

"No, not then."

"If he was with a group, didn't he have someone he knew who had a practice closer to the problem than orthopedic surgery?"

Cathy was getting scared and angry. "This is all so pointless. When we got to the hospital, they put him away. Something was wrong. Why pick on me?"

The therapist spoke again still looking at the papers in his lap. He addressed Chuck.

"This Dr. Winkler who examined you at Stockton, had you ever seen him before?"

"No."

"Did he have any reason to be prejudiced?"

"Maybe. We had a physician acquaintance in common, one who didn't care for me. Also, the minister whom my wife called talked to Dr. Winkler at great length before he saw me."

"What's that got to do with anything?" Cathy snapped. She was getting increasingly worried.

The therapist answered her. "It could have a lot to do with it, Cathy." Then he turned back to Chuck.

"Where's Dr. Winkler now? I don't remember hearing of him."

"Dr. Hill told me that Dr. Winkler is dead."

"What did he die of?"

"Dr. Hill didn't want to tell me what he died of. It took a lot of pressure to get the words out of him, but the cause of death, according to Dr. Hill, was Schizophrenic Paranoid."

The therapist raised his eyebrows as high as they would go. "That's the cause of death?"

"That is what I was told by Dr. Hill, yes."

"It was possible, then, that someone was giving away what they had?"

That was subtlely put, but the therapist had to be careful, there were professional ethics involved. What he had implied was that rather than face the problem in himself, Dr. Winkler was trying to see it in someone else and Chuck had been the "lucky" fellow.

"I don't remember ever hearing of that as a cause of death, have you, Chuck?"

"No, I haven't, never before. He had Amyotrophic Lateral Sclerosis. I'm surprised that that didn't take him first."

This was the opening for which Jane had been waiting. "Nobody can say all that, all that easily, unless they are a doctor. What kind of a doctor are you, Chuck?"

Chuck smiled, "I'm a pediatrician."

"Do you think that you are mentally ill?"

"No."

"Do you think you have ever been, excuse the word, crazy?"

"No."

She turned to Cathy. "Why do you think your husband is sick? You said you're here to help him."

"He's been confined in three different institutions, and had private treatments for months. What more do you want?"

The therapist didn't let her get away with that. "The hospital record is a mixed bag, Cathy. Let's stay away from it. Answer Jane's question in your own language. Why do you think that Chuck is sick?"

"Hallucinations. He thinks he had a wrestling match with Jesus Christ in the kitchen. That sounds pretty crazy to me."

Jane returned to the fray. "Are you a Christian?"

"Of course."

"Do you believe that Jesus appeared to Saul of Tarsus on the road to Damascus?"

"I suppose so."

"You suppose so! It's in the Bible plain as it can be. If Jesus can appear to one man after his resurrection, why not another?"

Cathy was getting angry and frustrated. Chuck knew that he could step in and stop it. All he had to do was to say he was sick enough to justify what happened. He didn't stop it, neither did the therapist, and Chuck wondered if they had both reached the same opinion. Cathy had seen more than one psychiatrist, and she had her share of unresolved problems. Nobody could get through to her by subtle means, anyway no one had succeeded up to this point. Maybe confrontation would do it, and this Jane seemed pretty tough. The therapist would have a critique on Cathy's condition from Hill as well as his paper work on Chuck. If he was willing to let things ride, Chuck decided to go along with him.

Cathy finally came up with a rebuttal. "It doesn't say that after Paul saw Christ, Paul couldn't get out of bed to get a drink of water."

"No, but he couldn't see either. He went blind."

The therapist interrupted again. "Chuck, do you know of any documentation, or of any trustworthy account of what happened to you having happened to anyone else?"

"Yes, in James' book VARIETIES OF RELIGIOUS EXPERIENCE there is a description of what I went through. It is described as happening to a Roman Catholic Saint.

"Then this experience is something that is recognized by the Catholic Church?"

"I think so. James implies it."

Jane resumed the battle. "What else made you think your husband was crazy?"

"He changed radically. He stopped wearing his glasses, stopped biting his nails."

Jane interrupted, "That's bad?"

Cathy continued, "He acted different, insisting on talking to people about religious things whether they wanted to hear it or not. He kept talking to patients about God and insisting on praying with them until he got thrown out of his medical group and ruined his practice."

John grinned. "Now we're getting down to the facts. He didn't ruin his practice. He ruined your spending money. His income went down."

"That's not important to me."

This obvious lie was greeted by derisive laughter from the whole group and Cathy flushed. "Well, I do object to being broke. I don't like it at all, and I don't like living in a small house with five children."

"How small is small?" Jane asked.

"It's only eighteen hundred square feet."

"Plus a two car garage?"

"Of course."

"Our house has twelve hundred square feet and we raised four kids in it. Where did you get that dress?"

"None of your business."

"Oh yes it is. You said you were broke. I know a little bit about clothes and how much they cost. I've worked in a department store. That dress cost a bundle and your shoes didn't come from the Salvation Army, and that nice tan doesn't come from scrubbing the kitchen floor. Broke, my left foot. Compared with everyone else in this room, you're living high on the hog and you're lying about a lot of things and wasting our time."

"I'm not the one who's wasting time. I'm not the one who is asking the questions. If you want to stop wasting time pick on somebody else."

That did it and Jane lowered the boom. "You are one thing else. You are the one real phoney in this room. Your beef with Chuck is that he quit making a lot of money. So you put him away where it would hurt until he'd change his mind and go back to being what you wanted him to be and it didn't work. Now I'll tell you why it didn't work. Your husband got solidly converted and he doesn't care about money. Now he cares about the Lord and about people and you can't stand to live with him. The contrast is too great."

There was dead silence in the room and Cathy was ashen. For the remainder of the session she would not say another word. She didn't say anything to Chuck as they drove back to Modesto, and she kept her silence until she was back with her children.

PART II

3 March 67
SACRAMENTO

When Chuck arrived the following week he arrived alone. Cathy had refused to come with him. When he entered the room there were greetings all around, questions about Cathy and her absence. The therapist admitted that the session had been rough, but he told Chuck to try to get Cathy back. She needed confrontation. There were solutions to her problems if she would pursue them.

The session started and Chuck sat through the first hour, making an occasional contribution, but generally feeling tired and despondent. The preceding week with Cathy had been unnerving. The tension at home had been extreme. He didn't know how much more he was going to be able to take. Cathy was angry all the way down to the bottom of her feet. She had said little, but the fires had smoldered.

At the end of the session's first hour, Chuck asked for the floor. He talked a little more about what he had been through, about what he was doing with his practice and about the hopelessness of his relationship with Cathy.

"You're sure she won't come back any more?" Jane asked.

"I'm sure. She has a wall built around her and you knocked a couple of bricks out of place and everyone could see through the wall a little. It let in a little light and she can't take that. To get well you have to admit you're sick and take the medicine."

The therapist asked if she would be willing to try more private therapy.

"No, I don't think so. Dr. Hill worked with her and with us for a number of sessions but every time he started to open the door a little she'd slam it shut. She cannot tolerate the possibility of being wrong. And that is a terrible way to live."

Chuck looked around the room before he continued. "Is there any reason in the minds of any of you for my coming to this group? Do any of you really think I need it? Because if you do I'll continue to come."

There was a long silence broken by the therapist. "Why don't you ask me?"

"All right, sir, I will. Should I continue to come?"

The therapist picked up Chuck's records from the small table beside him and wrote across the face of the top sheet. Then he signed his name followed by his M.D.

Chuck took the paper from the psychiatrist and read what had been written. Across the face of the top sheet of his report were the words, "Dramatically cured."

"Thank you. I guess that makes me a free man."

"It should."

Chuck walked back downstairs and out to his car. He sat in it for a while, saying a prayer of thanksgiving and quietly crying. When he had control of himself he started to drive back to Modesto. He drove in a leisurely manner. It was dark by the time he got home. He was surprised to see the house was dark.

He parked, walked to the front door and let himself in. When he turned on the light the room looked strangely bare. He walked through the house and almost everything personal was gone. There were few clothes, few toys, little evidence of any children. His wife's closet was empty. A further search showed that anything of value, the silverware, the silk screens they had brought from Japan, the paintings, anything that was worth money was no longer there. Some pictures with cheap frames and only sentimental value had not been taken.

Chuck went back into the living room, sat on the floor with his back to a wall and stared at nothing.

EPILOGUE

We had talked for hours. The bright light of day had turned to evening gloom. Outside, it had started to drizzle. All signs of Mt. Rainier were gone.

I had some questions. "Chuck, for a man who has been through what you have been through, you have a strange lack of bitterness, as a matter of fact, I don't sense any at all."

He smiled. "I used to be bitter, very bitter, but not any longer. You see, before I knew the Lord, I was stubborn, self-centered, conceited, hard-hearted, and anything else you want to say. God could not deal with me in an easy manner and get what He wanted. He had to put me through the wringer, and He did."

Chuck turned toward his desk. There was a Bible among the books that were stretched across it. He pulled it from its place and opened it as he talked. "I ran across this passage the other day, and it seems to apply to my situation. It's in the Prophet Hosea, the end of the fifth chapter, and it is God speaking to the Prophet. 'I will return again to my place, until they acknowledge their guilt and seek my face, and in their distress they seek me, saying, "Come, let us return to the Lord; for he has torn, that he may heal us; he has stricken, and he will bind up us." ' That seems to fit me exactly." He put the Bible back in its place.

I asked him another question. "After Cathy left, did you go on practicing medicine?"

"No, not for five years. The healing that Hosea talks about doesn't take place overnight. It took the Lord time to tear down, it took Him time to build back up. it was a while before I would consider medicine."

"When you did decide to go back to medicine, why did you come to this hospital and why do you stay? The 'turn over' in personnel must be high around here."

"The turn over is very high. It is a depressing place to work. It has to be, just because of what is here and what has to be done. I couldn't stay here without God's help and I wouldn't have come if He hadn't sent me."

"How can you know that God sent you?"

"I can show you that as we leave. It's time to go, anyway. We'll drive into town and get dinner."

We left his office and he locked the door. In the hallway that led to the rear entrance we met a couple of his colleagues. I was introduced and we exchanged pleasantries. I noticed something. Chuck was the only one who smiled.

At the back entrance of the hospital we found Chuck's car and got into it. He backed out of his parking space and drove around to the front of the hospital. As he did so, he began to talk again.

"When I decided that it was time to start practicing medicine, I wanted some kind of group practice where I would be working with and working under other doctors until I was back into the swing of things. This hospital was looking for a pediatrician, so I drove up here for a visit and an interview.

"The interview went well, but I really didn't know if I wanted to take the job even after it was offered. So, I wandered around the grounds for a while praying about it." The car swung around a curve and we could see the front entrance. Chuck pointed, "I was walking over there and I asked the Lord, 'If you want me here, show me some sign.' Let me show you what I found."

He parked the car and we climbed out into the drizzle. There was an old stone edifice still standing, one that had been part of the original construction of the earliest school. As we walked toward it I could see a brass plate embedded in the stone. There was just enough daylight left so that I could make out the words.

RAINIER STATE SCHOOL

"Inasmuch as ye have done it
unto one of the least of these
my brethren, ye have done
it unto me."

SAINT MATTHEW 25:40

Chuck said, "I read that, I knew who had said it, and I knew it was being said again to me. I took the job, and I'll be here until God moves me. His presence has made it far easier than I thought it would be."

We walked back to his car and got in. He continued talking. "I'm not a philospher nor a theologian, and there are a lot of things that I don't understand, but even if I don't understand them, I know how they work. For instance, this is a foggy and wintery evening. Not too pleasant, but I know that without it, there will be few flowers in the Spring. Why does God do things that way? I don't know, but I know the same thing applies spiritually. Suffering is followed by joy, if not in this life, then in the next, and I see this everywhere I look. Where there has been no real suffering, there is no real joy. I'm content to leave things in His hands."

He turned up the speed of his windshield wipers. The drizzle had become rain.

C. Brandon Rimmer